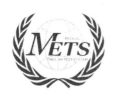

医护英语水平考试办公室
医护英语水平考试教研中心　组织编写

METS
测试与评析
（三级）
Level 3

主　编　饶　辉　龙　芸
（以下排名以姓氏笔画为序）

副主编　王　燕　李晓晖　杨发莉
　　　　雷　妍　戴月兰

编　者　王筱楠　陈继玲　何晓涛
　　　　吴灵梅　张　颖　穆东琴

U0360167

 南京大学出版社

图书在版编目（CIP）数据

METS 测试与评析. 三级 / 饶辉，龙芸主编. — 南京：
南京大学出版社，2018.12（2024.3 重印）
ISBN 978-7-305-20873-7

Ⅰ.①M… Ⅱ.①饶… ②龙… Ⅲ.①医学—英语—水
平考试—自学参考资料 Ⅳ.①R

中国版本图书馆 CIP 数据核字（2018）第 197709 号

出版发行　南京大学出版社
社　　址　南京市汉口路 22 号　　　　　邮　编　210093
书　　名　**METS 测试与评析（三级）**
　　　　　METS CESHI YU PINGXI(SAN JI)
主　　编　饶　辉　龙　芸
责任编辑　李　杰　刁晓静　　　　　编辑热线　025-83592123
照　　排　南京南琳图文制作有限公司
印　　刷　南京人文印务有限公司
开　　本　787×1092　1/16　印张 13.25　字数 380 千
版　　次　2018 年 12 月第 1 版　2024 年 3 月第 4 次印刷
ISBN 978-7-305-20873-7
定　　价　39.00 元

网址：http://www.njupco.com
官方微博：http://weibo.com/njupco
官方微信号：njupress
销售咨询热线：(025) 83594756

前　言

　　《METS 测试与评析》1—4 级系列丛书由医护英语水平考试办公室和医护英语水平考试教研中心组织编写,全国近 20 所各类医学院校 50 余名教师和专家参加编写和审稿工作。丛书对各级别 METS 考试的特点分别进行综述,其中相关试题严格按照 2017 年最新版《全国医护英语水平考试考试大纲》的要求进行设计,辅以较为详尽的分析和说明,并提供参考答案和作文范文,旨在帮助学生有效备考,顺利通过医护英语水平考试各级别的考试。本系列丛书既可供学生自主学习使用,又可以用作 METS 考试强化教材,也是英语教师开展 METS 考试研究的重要参考资料。

　　参加编写《METS 测试与评析》(三级)的教师包括:主编:饶辉(南京医科大学)、龙芸(贵州医科大学);副主编:王燕(滨州医学院/西安交通大学)、李晓晖(山东泰山护理职业学院)、杨发莉(贵州医科大学)、雷妍(贵州医科大学)、戴月兰(南京医科大学);编者:王筱楠(山东泰山护理职业学院)、陈继玲(中国药科大学)、何晓涛(贵州医科大学)、吴灵梅(山东泰山护理职业学院)、张颖(南京医科大学)、穆东琴(南京医科大学)。

目　录

医护英语水平考试（三级）考试综述

　　根据《全国医护英语水平考试考试大纲》(全新版)，METS 三级考试(笔试)由听力(Listening)、阅读(Reading)和写作(Writing)等三部分构成。考试时间为 120 分钟，成绩满分为 100 分。试卷结构，包括题型、题量、赋分、权重、考试时间等如下表所示：

	测试任务类型		为考生提供的信息	题目数量	原始分数	权重（%）	考试时间（分钟）
Ⅰ. 听力	Part One	信息匹配	短对话	5	5	30	30
	Part Two	信息判断	长对话	8	8		
	Part Three	多项选择	长对话	7	7		
	Part Four	填写信息	短文或长对话	5	5		
Ⅱ. 阅读	Part One	信息匹配	短文	10	10	45	60
	Part Two	多项选择	短文	7	7		
	Part Three	信息判断	短文	8	8		
	Part Four	补全短文	短文	5	5		
	Part Five	完形填空	短文	10	10		
Ⅲ. 写作		短文写作	提纲、情景等提示	1	15	25	30
总计				65＋1	80	100	120

　　为了帮助考生复习应考，我们将试卷的每个部分简述如下，内容包括考试要求、题型分析、真题简评、应试技巧介绍、备考策略等。

一、听力（Listening）

　　根据新大纲要求，听力测试由四个部分组成，共 25 题，主要考查考生理解口头信息的能力。本部分考试时间为 30 分钟，分数权重为 30%。

Part One　信息匹配

　　第一部分为 5 段临床对话选段(约 350 词)，要求考生根据听到的内容，辨识重要的或特定的信息,并将这些信息与选项中相应的病例描述相匹配。在给出的 6 个选项中,1 个为干扰项。每段对话选段之间有 3 秒钟的间隔供考生答题。录音播放两遍。

从近几年的真题来看,开篇的 5 段对话选段相对比较容易,内容主要是医生向患者解释病情或检查。对话选段中经常用到有关身体部位、疾病、症状、检查或治疗的医学词汇。近几年考题涉及的有关身体部位的词汇有 brain, heart, liver, pupil, spine, bladder, pancreas, humerus, intestine, extremities, blood vessel 等;有关疾病的词汇有 cold, cancer, angina, cystitis, fracture, hepatitis, melanoma, pneumonia, sleeplessness, tuberculosis, athlete's foot 等;有关症状的词汇有 tender, dilated, allergic, enlarged, cough, vomiting, anorexia, diarrhea, headache, dehydration, sore throat, infrequent urination, clear nasal discharge 等;有关检查的词汇有 EEG, X-ray, endoscopy 等;有关治疗的词汇有 cream, aspirin, dilator, steroid, diuretic, antibiotic, penicillin, medication, plaster cast, laser therapy 等。由此可见,该部分一般考查基本的医学词汇,但涉及的范围广。考试时,要充分利用播放指示语的时间迅速阅读各个选项,快速记住大意;之后,根据每段听力材料中重要的或特定的信息,将选项与之匹配。重要的信息一般会重复两到三次;特定的信息一般与选项中的信息一致。

Part Two 信息判断

本部分要求考生根据听到的一段长对话(约 400 词),对相关信息作出判断。有的信息是正确的,有的是错误的,有的对话中没有提及。这段录音播放两遍,每遍播完后有 3 秒钟的间隔供考生答题。

与第一部分相比,本部分的信息量较大,难度有所增加。从近年真题来看,医患之间的对话较为多见,也有对某个医学领域专家或学者的采访。医患之间的对话多发生在诊疗室,内容曾涉及 hepatitis, stomachache, low back pain 等常见疾病或症状。考题设计则多为对事实或细节的正误判断,如:"There is only one genotype of hepatitis C virus.""The patient has both diabetes and hepatitis."等;鲜有推理题或篇章题。

正误判断题在本质上是一种多项选择题,每道题有正确(True)、错误(False)以及没有提及(Not Given)等三个选项。其中,对所给句子作出正确的判断最为简单。答题时,听到的内容与题目相符,即可作出判断。对所给句子作出错误的判断稍难。所谓"错误"指的是题目中的陈述与听力材料中相应的内容不符。对所给句子作出未提及的判断最为困难。所谓"未提及"指的是听力材料没有涉及题目中的陈述。考试时,可用播放指示语的时间大致浏览所有选项,猜测对话的主题以及考点。播放对话时,逐个答题;对于第一次没有听清的事实或细节,第二次重点查听。

Part Three 多项选择

本部分要求考生根据听到的一段长对话(约 400 词),辨识重要或特定的细节内容,理解隐含的意义以及归纳中心思想,并从所提供的 3 个选项中选择一个最佳答案。录音播放两遍,每遍播完有 3 秒钟的间隔供考生答题。

第三部分和第二部分之间有不少相同之处,也有一些差异。相似之处在于,二者都是长对话,长度一致,且通常为医患之间的对话,偶见访谈;不同之处则在于第二部分的考题为事实题或细节题,仅需作出正误判断,而第三部分的考题不仅有事实题、细节题,还有推断题和归纳题,需选出正确答案。回顾近年真题,本部分的长对话曾涉及 stroke, arthritis, acute nephritis, breathing problems 等常见疾病或症状。如前所述,考题既有事实题、细节题,如:"What is the patient's chief complaint?"也有推断题和归纳题,如:"Which of the following can be inferred?"由此可见,第三部分有一定难度,需认真作答。考试时,要充分利用播放指示语的时间迅速阅读考题,猜测对话的主题以及考点。播放对话时,可以答题;对于第一次没有听清,无法作答的考题,第二次重点查听。对于推断题和归纳题,听时可在试卷相应考题的空白处稍做笔记。

Part Four　填写信息

本部分要求考生根据听到的一段长对话或短文(约 450 词),辨识重要的或特定的细节内容,并填写信息。这段录音播放两遍,每遍播完有 3 秒的停顿时间供考生答题。

与前三个部分相比,第四部分对考生的要求较高。考生不仅要听懂,还要写出重要的或特定的细节。从近几年的真题来看,本部分多为短文,内容曾涉及 breast cancer, chronic pain, CT-PET scan, colorectal cancer, primary health care, obsessive-compulsive disorder 等。考生看到的是信息不全的短文概要,需根据所听内容,补全概要。这部分有 5 个空格,要求填写 5 个单词,多为医学词汇,比如:iron, abuse, bowel, genetic, mental, maternal, injection, behavioral, secondary, depressive, defecation, biochemical, metastasis, metabolizing, colonoscopy, osteoarthritis, epidemiologist, physiotherapist, non-communicable, post-menopausal 等,也有少量普通词汇,比如:monitor, lifestyle, findings, strenuous 等。由此可见,多数单词较长,不易写对,少数单词比较简单。考试时,考生应在播放指示语时迅速浏览所给概要,猜测听力材料的话题和所缺内容。播放对话时,开始逐个答题。听到所缺内容后,不要急于全部记下,可用首字母、汉语或符号稍做笔记,以免因写已听到的信息而错过新信息。对于第一次没有听清的事实或细节,第二次重点查听。

学习建议:

三级听力试题有四个部分:信息匹配、信息判断、多项选择和填写信息。我们在前面对上述各部分的题型及解题技巧等作了简要说明。虽然熟悉题型和掌握技巧有助于提高答题的正确率,但是更重要的是平时的听力训练。没有持之以恒的练习,任何技巧都无济于事。因此,考生平时要多接触各类英语视听材料,如:TED(ideas worth spreading)、VOA、BBC、ABC news 等。如前所述,听力考试的前三部分基本是医患对话,涉及的内容广泛。备考时,应认真学习不同科室医生诊疗英语会话的结构和常用表达(包括如何询问主诉、病史、请患者配合检查、告知诊断结果以及治疗方案等);还应全面复习临床上常用的医学词汇,尽量做到听说读写"四会"。此外,第三部分听力材料也会从访谈中节选。考生平时可以多接触此类听力材料,如:《新英格兰医学杂志》官网上的访谈等。对于第四部分,考生应在平时重视单词的读音和拼写,方能正确填写所缺信息。总而言之,大量听力练习,辅以解题技巧才能提高听力部分的成绩。

二、阅读(Reading)

阅读测试由五个部分组成,主要考查考生理解书面信息的能力。这部分考试时间为 60 分钟,分数权重为 45%。

Part One 信息匹配

本部分考查考生理解医学短文(约 500 词)中重要信息以及归纳段落大意的能力。从近年真题来看,这部分一般为 5—7 段文字,内容涉及 paper medicine, health benefit plans, amyotrophic lateral sclerosis, gastroesophageal reflux disease, approach to breaking bad news, how to take vital signs before performing CPR 等。短文后面有两项考题:第一项考题考查考生归纳段落大意的能力;第二项考题则考查考生理解重要信息的能力。第一项考题中有 6 个选项,其中 1 个为干扰项。考生阅读相应段落后,总结其大意,并将这些信息与选项中相应的内容相匹配。有的段落有主旨句,位置在段首、段中或段末;有的段落没有主旨句,需要考生自己概括。阅读每一个段落、每一句话时,思考其大意,并分析每句话之间的关系;切忌力求读懂每个单词。一般来说,此项考题不难,易于得分。第二项考题也有 6 个选项,其中 1 个为干扰项。此项考题要求考生根据短文内容补全句子。答题时,先阅读所给句子,然后根据句子中的关键词(如:主语或谓语动词)从短文中寻找相关的内容。回顾历年真题,所填内容一般与医学相关,如:obese patients, lumbar puncture, motor neurons, muscle biopsy, medical records, emergency services, electronic case files, potential side effects 等。由于段落大意和重要信息不易快速识别,因此建议做题前略读全文,做题时认真阅读相应段落或句子。总的来说,本部分属于信息匹配而且干扰项较少,难度不大。

Part Two 多项选择

本部分考查考生理解医学短文(约 550 词)中明确或含蓄表达的重要信息的能力,以及归纳主旨大意的能力。题目要求考生在读懂全文的基础上,从每题所给的 4 个选项中选出最佳答案。

多项选择题被广泛用于国内外各级各类英语考试,如:雅思、托福、高考英语等,因此,METS 三级考试也采用了这种题型。从近几年真题来看,这部分内容涉及的话题比较广泛,如:Ebola infection, drug development, Parkinson's disease, transplanted bacteria, pregnancy and smoking 等,基本属于医学科普文章。这部分的细节题居多:有的考查考生理解明确的重要信息的能力,如:"According to the National Osteoporosis Foundation, how many American women suffer from osteoporosis?"有的考查考生理解隐含的重要信息的能力,如:"According to the passage, the research reported in *Science* demonstrates that _____."也有的考查考生理解文章主旨的能力,如:"The primary purpose of this passage is to _____."还有词汇理解题,如:"What does the word 'rodents'(in the last sentence of the 2nd paragraph) refer to?"由此可见,与信息匹配题相比,多项选择题覆盖的内容较为广泛,而且干扰项较多,具有一定难度。对于这种题型,考生可以先大致浏览考题,带着问题阅读短文。对于某一道题,找到短文中相对应的内容后,可以直接选出正确答案，也可以运用排除法、推理法等方法确定正确答案。

Part Three　信息判断

本部分考查考生理解医学短文（约400词）中明确或含蓄表达的重要信息的能力。题目要求考生在读懂全文的基础上，对给出的8个句子所表达的信息作出正确（True）、错误（False）或未提及（Not Given）的判断。

近几年真题中，这部分涉及的话题有 medicare，safety announcement，early menopause and later depression，acquisition of clinical skills，vaccine to prevent cholera，the use of stem cells for treating lung diseases 等。从考题来看，真题中仍以细节题居多，如："The pre-filled glass syringes may malfunction，break，or become clogged during the process of attempting to connect to needleless Ⅳ access systems"，"Postmenopausal depression has been offset by the use of hormone replacement therapy."等。

如前所述，正误判断题在本质上是一种多项选择题。与第二部分多项选择题相比，这种题型较为简单。这部分每道题只有 True，False 以及 Not Given 等三个选项。其中，对所给句子作出正确的判断最为简单。答题时，找到题目在文中相对应的句子或段落，仔细阅读即可。对所给句子作出错误的判断稍难。所谓"错误"指的是题目中的陈述与文中相应的内容不同。对所给句子作出未提及的判断最为困难。所谓"未提及"指的是无法在文中找到题目中的陈述。对于这部分考题，仔细阅读，不难得分。

Part Four　补全短文

本部分考查考生理解医学短文（约500词）篇章结构的能力。所给短文中缺少5个句子，文后有6个备选句子，要求考生根据全文主旨以及所缺句子上下文，选择合适的句子。

近几年的真题曾涉及 genes，narcolepsy，doctor-patient communication，flu and other viral infections，planning oncology clinic visits，importance of asking family members 等内容。所缺句子一般位于段中，也有在段末的，鲜有在段首的。所缺句子或长，如："When these pathogens spread throughout the body，they will inject their genetic material—comprised of RNA—inside of healthy cells，taking them over and replicating to form new viruses."或短，如："These proteins，they knew，are produced abundantly in the obese."对于正确作答，所缺句子的位置或长短不是首要的，最重要的是句子与上下文之间的逻辑关系。因此，考试时，应先对整篇文章有整体的理解，特别是各个段落之间的关系，之后根据所缺句子的上下文选择最合适的句子。与阅读部分其他考题相比，本部分考题难度较大，对考生的逻辑思维能力要求较高。

Part Five　完形填空

本部分通过一篇约400词的短文综合考查考生的语言理解及使用能力。所给短文被删掉10个单词。对于每个所缺词语，考生需在理解全文主旨以及所缺词语上下文的基础上，从4个选项中选出最佳选项填入空白处。

本部分题型为多项选择式完形填空，比开放式完形填空（不提供任何选项）简单一些，可综合考查考生的词汇、语法、篇章等不同语言层次的能力。最近几年的真题中，本部分的内容较为广泛,比如:vaccination, misuse of antibiotics, cluster of cancer cases, locating intramuscular injection sites, behavioral health screening in children, informed consent and the use of biospecimens in research 等。纵观近年真题,本部分多数考题考查考生根据上下文选择恰当词汇的能力,特别是与医学相关的名词、动词、形容词等,如:fever, episode, evaluate, incidence, carcinogen, in vitro, undiagnosed 等;也有一些题目考查语法或句子衔接。答题时,应先快速阅读全文,掌握文章主旨,然后根据主旨和上下文,逐个答题。第一遍作答时,如遇到无法短时完成的题目,可以暂时空着,继续答题。第二遍作答时,检查已完成的题目,完成未完成的题目。对于某一道题,根据全文主旨以及上下文,可以直接选出正确答案,也可以运用排除法、推理法等方法确定正确答案。

学习建议:

三级阅读部分由信息匹配、信息判断、多项选择、补全短文和完形填空等五个部分组成。如前所述,本部分题量是听力部分的两倍,权重高达 45%,是整个试卷中最重要的部分。阅读部分的成绩在一定程度上与能否通过考试密切相关。

如何提高阅读部分的成绩? 纵观历年真题,阅读部分涉及的话题十分广泛,包括疾病(如:Parkinson's disease, gastroesophageal reflux disease, amyotrophic lateral sclerosis 等),临床常规操作(如:approach to breaking bad news, how to take vital signs before performing CPR, acquisition of clinical skills 等),药品(如:drug development, misuse of antibiotics 等),医学研究成果(如:pregnancy and smoking, the use of stem cells for treating lung diseases 等)等。因此,平时应广泛涉猎相关知识,具备一定常识。阅读材料可为教材、报纸、杂志等。国内医学英语阅读类教材比较多,可选择人民卫生出版社出版的《医学专业英语—阅读分册》、南京大学出版社出版的《医学英语阅读教程》等。不少英文报纸杂志都有健康栏目,比如:*Reader's Digest*《读者文摘》,*Scientific American*《美国科学》,可在其官方网站阅读,非常方便。此外,还可以阅读世界卫生组织(WHO)、美国国立卫生研究院(the National Institutes of Health)等国外医疗机构网站上的内容。大量阅读不仅能够帮助我们增长医学知识,还能提高语言能力,特别是阅读能力。在大量阅读的基础上,可以利用高等教育出版社出版的《全国医护英语水平考试综合教程》及《全国医护英语水平考试应试指南》等全国医护英语水平考试系列用书,熟悉考试题型,掌握解题技巧。总而言之,大量阅读,辅以解题技巧才能提高阅读部分的成绩。

三、写作（Writing）

Part Six 写作

本部分考查考生书面表达的能力,要求考生根据试题所提供的信息撰写一篇约 150 词的短文。这部分考试时间为 30 分钟,分数权重为 25%。

本部分为命题作文,要求考生根据标题、提纲等给定的信息撰写短文。近几年真题的作文题目多为考生较为熟悉的,比如:what makes a good doctor/nurse, communication between doctors and patients, young people's unhealthy lifestyles must be changed, there should be a limit to the number of patients a doctor can see in one day 等。在理解题目的基础上,考生需要根据所给提纲构思作文的结构和具体内容。以 there should be a limit to the number of patients a doctor can see in one day 为例。给定提纲为"有必要限制每天门诊病人的数量"和"这样做的好处"。作文可以分成四段。第一段阐述观点:"有必要限制每天门诊病人的数量"。第二段列出对患者的好处。第三段阐述对医生的好处。第四段总结全文。语言要通顺、流畅、无语病。若能恰当使用排比、比喻、重复等常见的修辞手法,将为作文锦上添花。总而言之,作文的内容要切题、结构要清晰、语言要流畅。写作时,要尽量用英语思维,避免汉语的干扰。要想做到这点,平时就要加强阅读和写作训练。

学习建议:

写作是一项高级的语言活动,其重要性不言而喻。METS 四个级别均设有写作测试,考生应加强写作练习,提高写作能力。关于三级写作要求和技巧已有评述,下面再补充几点,供考生参考。

(1)一致性

一致性是英文写作的基本要求。句子内部、段落内部以及篇章内部均需保持一致性。句子的一致性指的是每个句子表达一个中心意思。从结构来讲,句子可简单(由一个分句构成),也可复杂(由多个分句构成),然而,从内容来讲,每个句子重点表达一个意思。同理,每个段落也要表达一个意思;每篇文章亦如此。写作时,首先要确定文章的中心意思,然后确定每个段落的大意,最后再斟酌每句话所表达的内容。为了保持文章一致性,审题后,不要提笔就写,要列出提纲或者打好腹稿。对于段落和句子一致性,需要专门练习。

(2)连贯性

连贯性亦为英文写作的基本要求。同一致性一样,句子内部、段落内部以及篇章内部均需保持连贯性。句子连贯性指的是句子各个成分之间有机连接。国内的英语学习者最常犯的错误就是用逗号连接两个或两个以上完整的英文句子。这种错误叫做"逗号粘连错误"。造成这种错误的主要原因可能是受汉语的影响。在汉语中,我们可以用逗号分隔两个句子,如:"据说苏州园林有一百多处,我到过的不过十多处。"然而,在英语中,逗号没有这样的用法。同理,段落内各个句子之间,以及文章的各个段落之间都应保持有机连接。段落内部的连贯性主要依靠衔接手段来实现。英语中常用的衔接手段是重复关键词或短语,使用同义词、代词,连接性表达以及某些句型(如:平行结构)。其中,最常用的是连接性表达。按照语义,连接性表达可分为递进(如:also, and, besides, equally, furthermore, in addition, moreover, what is more)、比较(如:compared with, in comparison with, in the same way/manner, likewise, similarly)、对比(如:although, but, conversely, however, in contrast, instead, nevertheless, on the contrary, whereas, while, yet)、列举(如:firstly, secondly, thirdly, finally, in the first place, last, to begin with, next, then)、让步(如:although it is true that, granted that, it may appear, it may be the case that)、举例(如:for example, for instance, to illustrate, such as, let us take the case of)、总结(如:in all, in brief, to summarize, in summary, in short, in conclusion, therefore, in a nutshell, on the whole, to sum up)、时间(如:after, afterwards, at first, at last, as long as, before, concurrently, first, finally, immediately, in the end, in the future, later, since, soon, subsequently, so far, somewhat earlier, thereafter, meanwhile, while)、结果(accordingly, as a result, as a consequence of, brought about by, consequently, contribute to, for that reason, hence, is due to, lead to, result in, thus)、重述(如:in other words，put simply，that is to say 等)、位置(如：above，behind，beyond，closer to，in the back，in front，nearby，to the left，to the right)等多类。段落之间遵从一定的逻辑顺序，例如：并列、递进、相反等。

综上所述，小到一个句子，大到一篇文章，都要保持一致性和连贯性。此外，若要做到"言之有物"，还需多读书、多观察、多思考。英文写作能力的提高不是一朝一夕的事情，需要"滴水穿石"的精神。只要坚持积累，不断练习，写作水平定会不断提高。

医护英语水平考试(三级)

模拟训练(一)

Medical English Test System (METS)
Level 3

Ⅰ Listening

Part One >>>>>>

 Questions 1—5

- You will hear five extracts from conversations taking place in different clinical departments.
- Choose which case each doctor is discussing from the list **A—F**.
- Use each letter **A—F** only once. There is one extra letter which you **DO NOT** need to use.
- Mark the corresponding letter on your **answer sheet**.
- You will hear each extract twice.

Doctor 1 [1]

Doctor 2 [2]

Doctor 3 [3]

Doctor 4 [4]

Doctor 5 [5]

A. The patient has an advanced eye tumor.

B. The patient is going to receive a brain CT.

C. The patient is anxious about the operation.

D. The patient has just finished his operation.

E. The patient has some problem with his stomach.

F. The patient will have an intravenous pyelogram.

Part Two >>>>>>

Questions 6—13

- You will hear a conversation between two doctors.
- For each of the following statements, decide whether it is **True (A)** or **False (B)**. If there is not enough information to answer **True (A)** or **False (B)**, choose **Not Given (C)**.
- Mark the corresponding letter on your **answer sheet**.
- You will hear the recording twice.

---

6. Dr. Jim is reluctant to discuss the patient's condition with Dr. Mary.
   A. True   **B.** False   **C.** Not Given

7. Mr. Alan Jameson is a frequent attender of Dr. Mary.
   A. True   **B.** False   **C.** Not Given

8. The pain of the patient came on about six weeks ago.
   A. True   **B.** False   **C.** Not Given

9. The patient's work has been affected by the pain.
   A. True   **B.** False   **C.** Not Given

10. Though depressed, the patient has no weight change.
    A. True   **B.** False   **C.** Not Given

11. The pain is accompanied by some tingling in his right hand.
    A. True   **B.** False   **C.** Not Given

12. Before he came to see the doctor, the patient had enjoyed good health.
    A. True   **B.** False   **C.** Not Given

13. The patient has been diagnosed with osteoarthritis.
    A. True   **B.** False   **C.** Not Given

Part Three >>>>>>

Questions 14—20

- You will hear a discussion among a supervising physician and two medical students.
- For questions **14—20**, choose the most appropriate answer.
- Mark the corresponding letter on your **answer sheet**.

- You will hear the discussion twice.

14. The common causes of asthma include the following EXCEPT _____.

    A. air   **B.** infection   **C.** irritants and allergies

15. Several studies show that the chances of developing asthma will be increased by _____.

    A. personality   **B.** diet   **C.** heredity

16. How many people died of asthma every year?

    A. Approximately 500.   **B.** Approximately 5,000. **C.** Approximately 50,000.

17. Which of the following is NOT thought to be the components of asthma attack?

    A. Swelling of the airways.

    B. Constriction of the muscles around the body.

    C. Inflammation.

18. Which of the following statements about acute severe asthma is true?

    A. It is responsive to routine therapy.

    B. Its attack may be slow, but the result is rapidly fatal.

    C. Patients will have difficulty in talking.

19. The treatment of acute severe asthma should be _____.

    A. immediate and aggressive

    B. accurate and balanced

    C. given under the permission of the patient

20. Monitoring of blood oxygen saturation should be performed as well as _____.

    A. arterial blood gas analysis

    B. monitoring of heart-beating

    C. monitoring of blood sugar

Part Four >>>>>>

Questions 21—25

- You will hear a speech on various contraceptive methods.
- Complete the notes. In each blank, write only one word.
- Write the answers on your **answer sheet**.
- You will hear the speech twice.

Notes:

There are different types of contraceptive pills that you need to think about and they all work differently:

- The (**21**) _____ which has a single hormone in it

  Be more careful about when you take it because it only has a three-hour gap in which it is safe.

- The combined pill with two types of hormones in it

  People have problems with both types of pills, for example, they get headaches or (**22**) _____ or put on weight and some people also have problems with their blood pressure.

- Coil

  We don't normally recommend this to women until they've had at least one child.

  If you do have any pelvic inflammatory diseases, it can be made worse, and it can increase the risk of (**23**) _____.

- The cap or diaphragm

  It doesn't involve any hormones.

  You do have to have it quite carefully fitted.

- Be sterilized or as it is sometimes called "have your tubes tied"

  This normally involves just a minor operation.

  It's a very, very reliable method. It has a very low failure rate.

  Its main drawback is that it should be regarded as being absolutely (**24**) _____.

- Coitus interruptus, an extremely unreliable method

- Condoms or sheaths, a safe and reliable method of contraception

  The main disadvantage is that they have to be put on during or shortly before intercourse.

  However, they do have the advantage of protecting against (**25**) _____ transmitted diseases.

II Reading

Part One >>>>>>

 Questions 26—35

• Read the following passage about general nutritional information.

General Nutritional Information

1 Making wise food choices early in life will help prevent health problems that can affect you later. It is reported that 8 of the 10 leading causes of death in America are directly related to what we eat and drink. Your eating habits, along with a smart exercise program, are crucial elements on the path to a healthier body and self.

2 Experts recommend limiting your fat intake to 30% of the total calories you consume per day. For a moderately active woman, you should consume approximately 2,000 calories and 65 grams of fat each day. For a moderately active man, you should consume approximately 2,500 calories and 80 grams of fat. If you want to lose weight, the equation is simple, eat less and exercise more. If you reduce your caloric intake by 500 calories per day, you will lose 1 pound per week. Alternatively, if you consume the same amount of calories, but increase your activity level to burn an additional 500 calories per day, you will also lose 1 pound per week. The easiest way to decrease the number of calories your body stores as fat is to not consume those calories in the first place; especially since it is much more difficult to burn calories once they are consumed. For weight loss it is recommended that you do not decrease your calorie and fat intake to any less than 1,200 calories and 40 grams of fat. Starvation diets or losing weight too fast can be dangerous.

3 A consistent pattern of daily physical activity and exercise is one of the healthiest habits you can get into. Studies have shown that physical activity tends to decrease with age, so now is the time to start. Walking to classes, taking stairs instead of elevators and becoming involved in sports and other physical activities are just a few of the many ways to develop a more active life-style. The time you spend on physical activity each day will also give your mind a much-needed break from its academic workout. And besides, exercise makes you feel wonderful, provided that you do not overdo it. So start slow, set goals for yourself, and get moving!

4 Vegetarianism is becoming increasingly popular among college students. It is estimated that 15% of the current college-age population in America is vegetarian. There are several different types of vegetarian diets, and each is chosen for a variety of reasons. Some people consider themselves vegetarian simply because they do not eat red meat. As far as nutritional recommendations for vegetarian diets, protein, iron and calcium can become an issue for those who do not consume animal products.

5 A healthy outlook about your body and appearance and how it relates to food and physical activity is very important for young adults. Self-destructive behaviors, which lead to eating disorders, such as eating a diet with too little fat or calories or embarking on a severe regime of physical activity, can have very harmful consequences to the health of your body and mind. Keep your mind and body in shape by treating them both with respect. A healthy self-image and realistic perception of yourself is one of the healthiest feats you can achieve.

 ## Questions 26—30

- Choose the most appropriate subheading from the list **A—F** for each paragraph.
- Use each letter **A—F** only once. There is one extra letter which you **DO NOT** need to use.
- Mark the corresponding letter on your **answer sheet**.

26. Paragraph 1 _____

27. Paragraph 2 _____

28. Paragraph 3 _____

29. Paragraph 4 _____

30. Paragraph 5 _____

A. Good nutrition is your choice
B. Keep balance between calorie intake and exercise
C. Fitness can be fun!
D. Growing trend of vegetarianism
E. Respect health
F. What do people usually expect from the high-profile sport events?

Questions 31—35

- Fill in each blank with the correct answer from the list **A—F**.
- Use each letter **A—F** only once. There is one extra letter which you **DO NOT** need to use.
- Mark the corresponding letter on your **answer sheet**.

31. It is reported that 80% of leading causes of death in America are directly related to _____.

32. To lose weight，two options are recommended：_____.

33. It is much more difficult to burn calories _____.

34. Vegetarian diets should contain protein，iron and calcium _____.

35. One of the healthiest feats you can achieve is _____ and realistic perception of yourself.

> **A.** once they are consumed
> **B.** instead of red meat
> **C.** a healthy self-image
> **D.** eat less and exercise more
> **E.** starvation diets
> **F.** what we eat and drink

Part Two >>>>>>

 Questions 36—42

- Read the following passage about a respiratory disease.
- Choose the best answer **A，B，C** or **D**.
- Mark the corresponding letter on your **answer sheet**.

COPD

COPD，or chronic obstructive pulmonary disease，is a <u>progressive</u> disease that makes its victim hard to breathe. COPD can cause coughing that produces large amounts of mucus (a slimy substance)，wheezing，shortness of breath，chest tightness，and other symptoms. Cigarette smoking is the leading cause of COPD. Most people who have COPD smoke or used to smoke. Long-term exposure to other lung irritants—such as air pollution, chemical fumes, or dust—also may contribute to COPD.

To understand COPD, it helps to understand how the lungs work. The air that you breathe goes down your windpipe into tubes in your lungs called bronchial tubes or airways. Within the lungs, your bronchial tubes branch into thousands of smaller, thinner tubes called bronchioles. These tubes end in bunches of tiny round air sacs called alveoli. Small blood vessels called capillaries run through the walls of the air sacs. When air reaches the air sacs, oxygen passes through the air sac walls into the blood in the capillaries. At the same time, carbon dioxide (a waste gas) moves from the capillaries into the air sacs. This process is called gas exchange. The airways and air sacs are elastic (stretchy). When you breathe in, each air sac fills up with air like a small balloon. When you breathe out, the air sacs deflate and the air goes out.

In COPD, less air flows in and out of the airways because of one or more of the following:

- The airways and air sacs lose their elastic quality.
- The walls between many of the air sacs are destroyed.
- The walls of the airways become thick and inflamed.
- The airways make more mucus than usual, which can clog them.

In the United States, the term "COPD" includes two main conditions—emphysema and chronic bronchitis. In emphysema, the walls between many of the air sacs are damaged. As a result, the air sacs lose their shape and become floppy. This damage also can destroy the walls of the air sacs, leading to fewer and larger air sacs instead of many tiny ones. If this happens, the amount of gas exchange in the lungs is reduced. In chronic bronchitis, the lining of the airways is constantly irritated and inflamed. This causes the lining to thicken. Lots of thick mucus forms in the airways, making it hard to breathe. Most people who have COPD have both emphysema and chronic bronchitis. Thus, the general term "COPD" is more accurate.

COPD develops slowly. Symptoms often worsen over time and can limit your ability to do routine activities. Severe COPD may prevent you from doing even basic activities like walking, cooking, or taking care of yourself. Most of the time, COPD is diagnosed in middle-aged or older adults. The disease isn't passed from person to person—you can't catch it from someone else. COPD has no cure yet, and doctors don't know how to reverse the damage to the airways and lungs. However, treatments and lifestyle changes can help you feel better, stay more active, and slow the progress of the disease.

36. The term "progressive" in the first paragraph can be defined as _____.

    A. having more and more irritability

    B. getting worse over time

C. appearing better over time

D. losing its natural quality

37. Which one is NOT the symptom of chronic obstructive pulmonary disease?

  A. Productive cough and wheezing.

  B. Wheezing and chest tightness.

  C. Shortness of breath and productive cough.

  D. Coughing with large amount of blood.

38. What is the normal pathway of air that you breathe into your lungs?

  A. Windpipe，bronchial tubes，bronchioles，alveoli.

  B. Bronchial airways，bronchioles，capillaries，air sacs.

  C. Windpipe，bronchioles，air sacs，capillaries.

  D. Air sacs，capillaries，bronchioles，windpipe.

39. Why does less air flow in and out of the airways in the chronic obstructive pulmonary disease?

  A. The elastic quality of the lungs is increasing beyond normal limit.

  B. There is less mucus to make the airways smoother.

  C. The inflammatory airways are becoming more and more narrowed.

  D. The gas exchange cannot occur between the walls of the airways and capillaries.

40. It can be inferred from the passage that _____.

  A. emphysema develops less advanced than chronic bronchitis

  B. chronic bronchitis is infrequently complicated by emphysema in most people

  C. there is ambiguity between emphysema and chronic bronchitis，thus COPD is more accurate

  D. emphysema is more difficult to treat than chronic bronchitis in most people who have COPD

41. Which is true about the treatments for COPD according to the passage?

  A. The damage to the airways and lungs can be reversed and cured by medicine.

  B. COPD is a kind of communicable disease，thus prevention and isolation is important.

  C. There is no cure for COPD but some ways to slow the progress of the disease.

  D. Lifestyle changes hold negative effect for patients with COPD.

42. Which one of the following statements is NOT true according to COPD?

  A. Cigarette smoking is the leading cause of COPD.

  B. COPD is a non-communicable disorder and has two conditions.

C. Middle-aged or older adults are more susceptible to COPD.

D. Doctors have the new approach to treat the damage of the airways.

Part Three >>>>>>

 ## Questions 43—50

- Read the following passage about the Ebola epidemic.
- For each of the following statements, decide whether it is **True (A)** or **False (B)**. If there is not enough information to answer **True (A)** or **False (B)**, choose **Not Given (C)**.
- Mark the corresponding letter on your **answer sheet**.

The Ebola Epidemic

On August 8, the World Health Organization (WHO) Director-General Margaret Chan declared the West Africa Ebola crisis a "public health emergency of international concern," triggering powers under the 2005 International Health Regulations (IHR).

Ebola virus disease (EVD) has 3 species of human significance: Zaire, Sudan, and Bundibugyo. The West Africa outbreak is from a new strain of the Zaire species, with a reported case-fatality rate of 55%. Infection can cause fever, vomiting, diarrhea, and generalized bleeding as well as death.

Fruit bats likely carry Ebola virus, with humans infected by close contact with infected body fluids and "bushmeat" of primates, forest antelope, wild pigs, and bats. Human-to-human transmission occurs only by close contact with infected body fluids. Importantly, no airborne transmission between humans has been demonstrated. Early EVD symptoms are similar to those of malaria and typhoid fever—as well as endemic hemorrhagic fevers such as Lassa—rendering symptomatic differential diagnosis difficult.

Before the current outbreak began in December 2013, West Africa had no recorded Ebola deaths. Yet this outbreak is the largest, with the crisis worsening. As of August 8, WHO reported 1779 Ebola cases, with 961 deaths. Cases were first reported in Guinea on March 23, followed by Liberia, Sierra Leone, and Nigeria (due to an infected airline passenger from Liberia). Of greatest concern is the potential urban spread, including capital cities. Previously Ebola was concentrated in rural areas, where the public health response was sufficiently rapid to prevent spread to populated cities.

Since 1976 more than 15 Ebola outbreaks have erupted in sub-Saharan Africa, yet therapeutic options remain undeveloped. There are no licensed vaccines or specific antivirals or immune-mediated treatments for ill patients or for postexposure prophylaxis. The US National Institutes of Health is supporting the first phase clinical trial of a new prototype experimental vaccine which is expected to begin in September 2014.

Fueling disquiet about global justice, 2 US aid workers infected in Liberia were treated with an experimental anti-Ebola antibody prior to being transported to Atlanta. This serum had been previously used only in nonhuman primates. Even though the serum's safety and efficacy remain unknown, it sparked an international controversy. Should US workers receive a drug in extremely scarce supply when Africans are affected in far greater numbers? Balanced against this sense of injustice is the ethical concern of administering an experimental drug to African patients that has not undergone any safety testing in humans.

On August 11, WHO convened an expert committee to assess the bioethical implications of withholding or providing early access to experimental treatments. If a scarce treatment offers benefits to patients, the ethical question is who should have priority access? Society, for example, owes a duty to health workers who place themselves at heightened risk. Other ethical considerations could be granting priority to patients most likely to benefit, as well as targeting the drug to prevent spread in hospitals or the community. Moreover, who should decide whether an experimental treatment should be administered? Liberian officials apparently did not approve the use of an investigational drug administered in their territory. National leaders also would need to be part of future decision making processes for allocating scarce vaccines and medications.

43. International Health Regulations was declared in the West Africa.

    A. True   **B.** False   **C.** Not Given

44. The West Africa Ebola outbreak is from a new strain with 55% case-fatality rate.

    A. True   **B.** False   **C.** Not Given

45. Social contact with infected people has been demonstrated as an important way of transmission.

    A. True   **B.** False   **C.** Not Given

46. Both rural and urban areas in West Africa have been involved in Ebola outbreak.

    A. True   **B.** False   **C.** Not Given

47. No effective vaccines are available for afflicted individuals or for postexposure prevention.

    A. True   **B.** False   **C.** Not Given

48. The experimental anti-Ebola antibody can be administered by African patients.

    A. True   **B.** False   **C.** Not Given

49. Two US aid workers infected in Liberia have recovered after treatment.

    A. True   **B.** False   **C.** Not Given

50. A great number of ethical questions need to be solved by WHO and national leaders together.

    A. True   **B.** False   **C.** Not Given

Part Four   >>>>>>

 ## Questions 51—55

- Read the following passage about aspirin overdose. Five sentences have been removed from the passage.
- Fill in each blank with the most appropriate sentence from the list **A—F**. There is one extra sentence which you **DO NOT** need to use.
- Mark the corresponding letter on your **answer sheet**.

What Should I Do about an Aspirin Overdose?

Aspirin overdose is an extremely serious and potentially life-threatening condition and there are two forms of which people should be aware. In acute aspirin poisoning a person takes far more than the recommended (in an adult 20,325 mg tablets) dosage, causing immediate poisoning. Another form of aspirin overdose is called chronic overdose and occurs when people take aspirin regularly. Especially in hot conditions, dehydration may result in residual amounts of aspirin not cleared properly from the body, and this can cause toxicity. **(51)** _____

The regular dose of aspirin for most adults is 325-650 mg every four to six hours. In children, aspirin is not recommended, though some kids with heart conditions may be on very low dose amounts to prevent blood clotting. **(52)** _____ For most kids, using this medication is not advisable because of the risk of developing certain conditions like Reye's syndrome.

Most cases of acute aspirin overdose are intentional, and there are several symptoms people may recognize that can occur within a few hours of the overdose. In acute overdose, people may have extreme stomach pain, nausea and/or vomiting. If the amount taken is very high other symptoms like ringing in the ears, dizziness or drowsiness, hyperactive behavior, seizures and coma can be present. People might recognize signs of chronic aspirin overdose if a person is fatigued, has a mild fever, is breathing rapidly or has a fast heartbeat, and even the person acts confused or faints.

(53) _____ When people suspect overdose they should call emergency services right away and try to keep the person who has overdosed calm. They should not offer food or water to that person, and it is not advisable to induce vomiting, which may do more harm than good. In most cases, people should wait for emergency services to arrive instead of attempting to take an overdose victim to the emergency room.

One of the difficulties with aspirin overdose is that there is no immediate antidote to it. In the hospital, people may be given charcoal, may be watched for developing symptoms, and may be required for dialysis to remove aspirin from the blood stream. There is no adequate home treatment that can replace hospital care, but even hospital care may sometimes be ineffective if the overdose has been ignored for several hours.

(54) _____ If they know the amount taken, the time the aspirin was taken, and the approximate weight and height of the overdose victim, this is great information to give to a dispatch worker. It isn't always possible to know this, but whatever extra information be given may prove helpful.

For parents, a special caution exists. Many companies still make forms of baby aspirin that are chewable. (55) _____ If there are adults (or kids with heart defects) who use the chewable form, keep these medications far out of reach of other children. An alternative is to use adult low dose aspirin, which is a small easy-to-swallow pill that doesn't have an attractive taste. In either case, this medication and all others should not be anywhere near children.

A. The chronic form is usually more likely in those people who take aspirin therapy and who have poor kidney function.

B. When people call emergency services, they can help greatly by having some information on hand.

C. Both types of aspirin overdose are medical emergencies and need immediate medical attention.

D. Low-dose aspirin is usually approximately 80 mg per day, and may be sold as low dose or "baby" aspirin.

E. These tend to taste good to kids and make aspirin overdose more likely.

F. They point out that aspirin overdose in baby patients is a normal part of the treatment.

Part Five >>>>>

 Question 56—65

- Read the following passage about laser eye surgery.
- Fill in each blank with the correct choice **A, B, C** or **D**.
- Mark the corresponding letter on your **answer sheet**.

Laser Eye Surgery

For many people, laser eye surgery can correct their vision so they no longer need glasses or (**56**) _____ lenses. Laser eye surgery reshapes the cornea, the clear front part of the eye. This changes its focusing power. There are different types of laser eye surgery. LASIK—laser-assisted in situ keratomileusis—is one of the most common. Many patients who have LASIK end up with 20/20 (**57**) _____.

The surgery should take less than 30 minutes. You will lie on your back in a reclining chair in an exam room containing the laser system. The laser system includes a large machine with a microscope (**58**) _____ to it and a computer screen. A numbing drop will be placed in your eye, the area around your eye will be cleaned, and an instrument called lid speculum will be used to hold your eyelids open.

Your doctor may use a laser keratome (a laser device), instead of a mechanical microkeratome (a blade device), to cut a flap on the cornea. If a laser keratome is used, the cornea is flattened with a clear plastic plate. Your vision will (**59**) _____ and you may feel the pressure and experience some discomfort during this part of the procedure. Laser energy is focused (**60**) _____ the cornea tissue, which creates thousands of small bubbles of gas and water that expand and connect to separate the tissue underneath the cornea surface, creating a flap. The plate is then removed.

You will be able to see, but you will experience (**61**) _____ degrees of blurred vision during the rest of the procedure. The doctor will then lift the flap and fold it back on its hinge, and dry the exposed tissue.

The laser will be positioned over your eye and you will be asked to stare at a light. This is not the laser used to remove tissue from the cornea. This light is to help you keep your eye fixed on one spot (**62**) _____ the laser comes on.

When your eye is in the correct position, your doctor will start the laser. At this point in the surgery, you may become aware of new sounds and smells. The pulse of the laser makes a ticking sound. As the laser (**63**) _____ corneal tissue, some people have reported a smell similar to burning hair. A computer controls the amount of laser energy delivered to your eye. Before the start of surgery, your doctor will have programmed the computer to vaporize a particular amount of tissue based on the (**64**) _____ taken at your initial evaluation. After the pulses of laser energy vaporize the corneal tissue, the flap is put back into position.

A shield should be placed over your eye at the end of the procedure as protection, since no stitches are used to hold the flap in place. It is important for you to wear this shield to prevent you from rubbing your eye and putting pressure on your eye while you sleep, and to protect your eye from (**65**) _____ being hit or poked until the flap has healed.

56. A. contact   **B.** artificial   **C.** hidden   **D.** concealed

57. A. power   **B.** degree   **C.** vision   **D.** eye

58. A. clipped   **B.** attached   **C.** fastened   **D.** implemented

59. A. clear   **B.** improve   **C.** blur   **D.** flag

60. A. over   **B.** on   **C.** inside   **D.** outside

61. A. additive   **B.** agonizing   **C.** flexible   **D.** fluctuating

62. A. once   **B.** before   **C.** until   **D.** since

63. A. screens   **B.** scrapes   **C.** implants   **D.** removes

64. A. assessments   **B.** evaluations   **C.** estimations   **D.** measurements

65. A. frequently   **B.** consequently   **C.** accidentally   **D.** undoubtedly

III Writing

Question 66

- Write about the following topic.

  Now, seeing a doctor is still a difficult and expensive affair in China. What are the causes behind this phenomenon? And what can be done to make the high-quality healthcare service accessible and affordable to ordinary people?

- Write an essay of no less than 150 words on your **answer sheet.**

医护英语水平考试(三级)

模拟训练(二)

Medical English Test System (METS)
Level 3

Ⅰ Listening

Part One >>>>>>

 Questions 1—5

- You will hear five extracts from conversations taking place in different clinical departments.
- Choose which case each doctor is discussing from the list **A—F**.
- Use each letter **A—F** only once. There is one extra letter which you **DO NOT** need to use.
- Mark the corresponding letter on your **answer sheet**.
- You will hear each extract twice.

Doctor 1 1	**A.** The patient is receiving a neurological examination of arms and legs.
Doctor 2 2	**B.** The patient suffered from appendicitis and may need an operation.
Doctor 3 3	**C.** The patient has a swollen ankle and needs a support bandage.
Doctor 4 4	**D.** The patient needs some medication to deal with problems of blood pressure and chest pain.
Doctor 5 5	**E.** The patient has to be hospitalized and isolated.
	F. The baby patient was preterm and had an infection and jaundice.

Part Two >>>>>>

Questions 6—13

- You will hear a conversation between the student nurse Barbara and her instructor, Mrs. Baker.
- For each of the following statements, decide whether it is **True (A)** or **False (B)**. If there is not enough information to answer **True (A)** or **False (B)**, choose **Not Given (C)**.
- Mark the corresponding letter on your **answer sheet**.
- You will hear the recording twice.

---

6. Nurse Barbara is taking care of the patient in Room 322 Bed 2.
   A. True **B.** False **C.** Not Given

7. The patient received an operation on the stomach in the morning.
   A. True **B.** False **C.** Not Given

8. The patient had a laparoscopic cholecystectomy.
   A. True **B.** False **C.** Not Given

9. The post-operative care for open cholecystectomy and laparoscopic cholecystectomy is different.
   A. True **B.** False **C.** Not Given

10. Laparoscopic cholecystectomy has replaced open cholecystectomy as the first choice of treatment for gallstones.
    A. True **B.** False **C.** Not Given

11. The focus of care for post-operative patients includes pain, incision care, vital signs, circulation and perfusion.
    A. True **B.** False **C.** Not Given

12. It is very important to help the post-operative patient cough effectively because coughing can help reduce the chance of getting pneumonia.
    A. True **B.** False **C.** Not Given

13. Coughing can help contract the lungs and clear the airway.
    A. True **B.** False **C.** Not Given

Part Three >>>>>>

 ## Questions 14—20

- You will hear a ward team meeting among four nurses discussing a patient with stroke.
- For questions **14—20**，choose the most appropriate answer.
- Mark the corresponding letter on your **answer sheet**.
- You will hear the discussion twice.

---

14. The patient Lidia is _____.

    A. a 60-year-old Russian lady living with her daughter

    B. a 70-year-old American lady living with her husband

    C. an 80-year-old Russian lady living alone

15. What is the main problem of Lidia?

    A. She had a heart disease.

    B. She had a stroke.

    C. She suffered from diabetes and hypertension.

16. When was Lidia sent to the hospital?

    A. Several hours after the onset of the stroke.

    B. Immediately after the onset of the stroke.

    C. Several days after the onset of the stroke.

17. What is Lidia's main goal?

    A. Staying at the hospital.

    B. Going back to her own home.

    C. Going to her daughter's home.

18. What day is the home assessment booked for?

    A. Tuesday，6th June.

    B. Friday，9th June.

    C. Monday，12th June.

19. Where is Lidia going to stay when she first gets out of the hospital?

    A. She's going to stay with her daughter.

    B. She's going to a nursing home.

    C. She's going to her own home.

20. Which of the following about Lidia's condition is true?

    A. Lidia has lost her vision on the right.

  B. Lidia still has some tongue and lip weakness.

  C. Tina has already referred Lidia to a Speech Therapist.

Part Four >>>>>>

 Questions 21—25

- You will hear a speech on the prostate removal.
- Complete the notes below by filling each space **21—25** with a single word.
- Write the answers on your **answer sheet**.
- You will hear the speech twice.

Notes:

 In older men it is quite common for the prostate to (**21**) _____ and cause the symptoms.

 What we need to do:

- Some drugs which may help

 I don't think the drugs will help in your case.

- Before the operation

 a few tests like blood and urine tests, heart tracing, a chest X-ray and sometimes an IVP, (**22**) _____ pyelogram

 type of (**23**) _____—a general when you would be completely asleep or an epidural which only numbs the lower part of your body

- Two ways of removing the prostate

 by operating after inserting a (**24**) _____ through the penis or by making a cut in the lower abdomen

- After the operation

 Your urine would be drained by a tube called an (**25**) _____ catheter.

 You'll also have a tube in your arm called IV which may supply you with saline or blood.

 Start drinking large quantities of fluid after the operation.

 Stool softener to avoid constipation.

 Slightly changed sex life.

Ⅱ Reading

Part One ＞＞＞＞＞

 Questions 26—35

• Read the following passage about yawn.

Yawn

1 We do know lots of interesting things about yawning: you start yawning in uterus; you yawn when you're aroused; and more than half of you will yawn if you see someone else yawn. While fatigue, drowsiness or boredom easily bring on yawns, scientists are discovering there's more to yawning than most people think. Not much is known about why we yawn or if it serves any useful function, and very little research has been done on the subject. However, there are several theories about why we yawn.

2 Scientists propose that our bodies induce yawning to draw in more oxygen and remove a buildup of carbon dioxide. This theory helps explain why we yawn in groups. Larger groups produce more carbon dioxide, which means our bodies would act to draw in more oxygen and get rid of the excess carbon dioxide. However, if our bodies make us yawn to draw in needed oxygen, wouldn't we yawn during exercise?

3 Some think that yawning began with our ancestors, who used yawning to show their teeth and intimidate others. An offshoot of this theory is the idea that yawning developed from early man as a signal for us to change activities. Another speculated reason for yawning is the desire to stretch one's muscles. Yawns are often accompanied by the urge to stretch. Prey animals must be ready to physically exert themselves at any given moment. There have been studies that suggest yawning, especially psychological "contagious", may have developed as a way of keeping a group of animals alert. If an animal is drowsy or bored, it may not be as alert as it should to be prepared to spring into action. Therefore, the "contagious" yawn could be an instinctual reaction to a signal from one member of the "herd" reminding the others to stay alert.

4 A more recent theory proposed by researchers is that since people yawn more in situations where their brains are likely to be warmer—tested by having some subjects breathe through their noses or press hot or cold packs to their foreheads—it's a way to cool down their brains. In 2007, researchers, including a professor of psychology, from the University of Albany proposed that yawning may be a means to keep the brain cool. Mammalian brains operate best within a narrow temperature range. In two experiments, they demonstrated that both subjects with cold packs attached to their foreheads and subjects asked to breathe strictly nasally exhibited reduced contagious yawning when watching videos of people yawning.

5 Recent studies show contagious yawning may be linked to one's capacity for empathy. In one study, autistic and non-autistic children were shown videos of people yawning and people simply moving their mouths. Both groups of kids yawned the same amount when viewing the video of people moving their mouths. But the non-autistic kids yawned much more frequently than those with autism when watching people really yawning. Since autism is a disorder that affects a person's social interaction skills, including the ability to empathize with others, the autistic kids' lack of yawning when watching others do so could indicate they're less empathetic. The study also found the more severe a child's autism, the less likely he or she was to yawn.

Questions 26—30

- Choose the most appropriate subheading from the list **A—F** for each paragraph.
- Use each letter **A—F** only once. There is one extra letter which you **DO NOT** need to use.
- Mark the corresponding letter on your **answer sheet**.

26. Paragraph 1 _____

27. Paragraph 2 _____

28. Paragraph 3 _____

29. Paragraph 4 _____

30. Paragraph 5 _____

  A. The physiological explanation

  B. Why do we yawn?

  C. Contagious yawning and empathy

  D. The brain-cooling hypothesis

  E. Various possible situations to occur

  F. The evolution theory

Questions 31—35

- Fill in each blank with the correct answer from the list **A—F**.
- Use each letter **A—F** only once. There is one extra letter which you **DO NOT** need to use.
- Mark the corresponding letter on your **answer sheet**.

31. One of the interesting things about yawning is that we start yawning _____.

32. The reason why we yawn easily at meeting may be that our body need inhale more oxygen and _____.

33. The "contagious" yawn could be a(n) _____ to a signal from one member of the prey animals reminding the others to stay alert.

34. Researchers including a psychologist proposed that yawning is used for _____ within a narrow range.

35. Contagious yawning don't frequently occur _____ since they are less empathetic.

> **A.** exhale excessive carbon dioxide
> **B.** in non-autistic kids
> **C.** regulation of brain temperature
> **D.** instinctual reaction
> **E.** in autistic children
> **F.** before we are born

Part Two >>>>>>

 Questions 36—42

- Read the following passage about obstructive sleep apnea.
- Choose the best answer **A, B, C** or **D**.
- Mark the corresponding letter on your **answer sheet**.

Obstructive Sleep Apnea

Your spouse says your snoring is driving her nuts. You wake up feeling unrested and irritable. These are common signs that you may have obstructive sleep apnea (OSA), a sleep disorder that—left untreated—can take its toll on the body and mind. Untreated OSA has been linked to high blood pressure, heart attacks, strokes, car accidents, work-related accidents and depression. With sleep apnea, your breathing pauses multiple times during sleep. The pauses can last from a few seconds to minutes and can occur more than five times per hour, to as high as 100 times per hour (Fewer than five times per hour is normal.). Sometimes when you start breathing again, you make a loud snort or choking sound.

Obstructive sleep apnea, the most common type, is caused by a blockage of the airway, usually when the soft tissue in the back of the throat collapses. The less common form, central sleep apnea, happens if the area of your brain that controls breathing doesn't send the correct signals to your breathing muscles.

Sleep apnea is almost twice as common in men as it is in women. Other risk factors include: being overweight, being over age 40, smoking and so on. Children also get sleep apnea, most commonly between ages 3 and 6. The most common cause is enlarged tonsils and adenoids in the upper airway.

Polysomnogram (PSG) is the most common sleep study for sleep apnea and often takes place in a sleep center or lab to record brain activity, eye movement, blood pressure and the amount of air that moves in and out of your lungs.

The first line of defense can be behavioral. Weight loss may go a long way toward improving OSA. It may also help by stoping using alcohol or medicines that make you sleepy, because they can make it harder for you to breathe.

The most common treatment is a Continuous Positive Airway Pressure (CPAP) machine. CPAP use mild air pressure to keep your airways open. The air is delivered through a mask that fits over your nose and mouth, or only your nose.

CPAP is not the only medical device approved for treatment of OSA. On May 1, 2014, Food and Drug Administration (FDA) approved the first implanted medical device for the treatment of this disorder. The Inspire Upper Airway System (UAS) is intended for consumers with moderate to severe OSA who have specific characteristics (a Body Mass Index under 32 and the absence of complete collapse in the back of the throat) and were not helped by a CPAP device, or could not tolerate the CPAP treatment. The Inspire device is surgically implanted below the collarbone and works with electrical impulses to stimulate the patient's tongue muscles and keep airways open.

The Inspire UAS consists of an electrical impulse generator, with leads and sensors that stimulate the nerve that controls the tongue and that senses the patient's breathing.

After the surgical site has healed (about a month), the physician turns the unit on and sets up the pulse generator. Patients may need to undergo one or more sleep studies before the UAS configuration is optimized for use. The patient turns the system on before going to sleep and off upon waking, using a remote control.

36. What is the meaning of the Greek word "apnea" in obstructive sleep apnea?

    A. Breakout.   **B.** Without breath.

    C. Dysfunction.   **D.** Without regulation.

37. Which one of the breathing pause during sleep is considered as normal?

    A. More than ten seconds.   **B.** Not less than ten minutes.

C. Ten times per hour.　　**D.** Four times per hour.

38. What is the cause of obstructive sleep apnea?

　　A. Enlarged tonsils and adenoids.

　　B. Paralysis of respiratory center in the brain.

　　C. Collapses of soft tissue of the throat.

　　D. Hypertension and heart attacks.

39. Who is more susceptible to sleep apnea?

　　A. Non-smoking and young female.

　　B. Obese older smoking male.

　　C. Male and female with BMI above 32.

　　D. Teenagers and young adults.

40. Which is NOT belonging to behavioral change for treatment of OSA?

　　A. Early to bed and early to rise.

　　B. Giving up alcohol.

　　C. Losing weight.

　　D. Withdrawing of sleeping pills administration.

41. It can be inferred from the passage that _____.

　　A. FDA prefers the Inspire UAS to CPAP machine because of its cost

　　B. as a noninvasive procedure，CPAP treatment has something in common with the Inspire UAS

　　C. the Inspire UAS treatment is more expensive than CPAP treatment

　　D. the Inspire UAS treatment is a kind of invasive procedure

42. Which of the following statements is true according to the passage?

　　A. Obstructive sleep apnea is less common than central sleep apnea.

　　B. Sleep apnea is as common in men as it is in women and children.

　　C. Not all OSA patients are candidates for Inspire UAS treatment.

　　D. The CPAP should be turned on before sleeping and off upon waking.

Part Three ≫≫≫≫

 ## Questions 43—50

- Read the following introduction of program provided by RMIT University.
- For each of the following statements，decide whether it is **True（A）** or **False（B）**. If there is not enough information to answer **True（A）** or **False（B）**，choose **Not Given（C）**.
- Mark the corresponding letter on your **answer sheet**.

PATHOLOGY TESTING

C5283 Diploma of Laboratory Technology (Pathology Testing)

Duration: 2 years

www. rmit. edu. au/programs/c5283

City campus

The Diploma of Laboratory Technology (Pathology Testing) will give you the practical skills and knowledge to pursue a technical career in pathology laboratories and hospitals.

As a medical laboratory technician or medical laboratory assistant, you will conduct routine laboratory tests for pathologists, microbiologists/bacteriologists, biochemists, clinical chemists, pharmacologists and veterinarians.

Working under supervision, you may examine micro-organisms or changes in cells and tissues, or perform chemical analyses of blood and other body fluids. You may also assist in performing experiments for research into biochemical or genetic processes.

Class sizes are small and the staff-to-student ratio in laboratories allows opportunities for individual teaching. Teachers have extensive industry experience and expertise and maintain close links with colleagues in the industry. RMIT has long been recognized by the pathology industry as providing quality training in the field.

Working with industry

You will undertake 20 days of work experience during the second year, organized by RMIT. This provides you with an opportunity to gain a greater understanding of the industry and to develop your laboratory skills in an area that also require teamwork, attention to quality control and working to timelines.

You may be placed in a variety of work environments, ranging from small research laboratories to large pathology companies.

What you will study

Year one

The first year provides you with a foundation in chemistry, maths, biology, scientific communication, computing, biochemistry and occupational health and safety.

You will learn general laboratory skills such as microscopy, aseptic techniques, chemistry techniques and the use of laboratory instruments. Labs have latest industry standard equipment and there is ample opportunity for you to gain hands-on experience.

In chemistry you will become skilled at preparing solutions that meet strict quality control standards. You will use specialized equipment, and learn to work safely with potentially dangerous chemicals.

Year two

The second year involves more specialized study in the major diagnostic areas relevant to a pathology lab. These include haematology, microbiology, histology and clinical chemistry, as well as quality assurance.

You will learn the skills to undertake blood counts, test levels of chemicals in blood, identify bacteria using a microscope and culture methods, as well as how to prepare thin slices of liver and other tissues to examine microscopically. All of these tests aid in the diagnosis of all types of diseases.

Teaching methods

Classes are taught in a combination of lecture, workshop, practical and laboratory sessions.

Career outlook

There is a high demand for technicians to work in pathology laboratories in both public hospitals and large private pathology providers such as Gribbles, Dorevitch and Melbourne Pathology.

Professional recognition

Students are eligible for student membership of the Australian Society for Microbiology and the Australian Institute of Medical Laboratory Scientists, and upon graduation are eligible for associate membership.

Pathways

Graduates of the Diploma of Laboratory Technology (Pathology Testing) who are successful in gaining a place are eligible to apply for exemptions of up to one year (96 credit points) from the following programs:

Bachelor of Applied Science (Laboratory Medicine)

Bachelor of Biomedical Science (Pharmaceutical Science)

Bachelor of Science (Biotechnology)

43. Pathology testing is concerned with various tests aiding in the diagnosis of various types of diseases.

    A. True   **B.** False   **C.** Not Given

44. Pathology laboratories in medical universities have great demand for technicians.

    A. True   **B.** False   **C.** Not Given

45. Work experience is arranged in the whole second year in small research laboratories.

    A. True   **B.** False   **C.** Not Given

46. Opportunities for individual teaching are guaranteed by small class size and staff-to-student ratio in laboratories.

    A. True   **B.** False   **C.** Not Given

47. Students should finish all courses when they apply for exemptions from final examination.

A. True   **B.** False   **C.** Not Given

48. The study of the first year involves both the foundational and specialized subjects.

    A. True   **B.** False   **C.** Not Given

49. Graduates of the Diploma of Laboratory Technology should know how to prepare thin slices of liver and other tissues to examine microscopically.

    A. True   **B.** False   **C.** Not Given

50. All students are the members of the Australian Society for Pathology.

    A. True   **B.** False   **C.** Not Given

Part Four >>>>>>

Questions 51—55

- Read the following passage about placebo effect. Five sentences have been removed from the passage.
- Fill in each blank with the most appropriate sentence from the list **A—F**. There is one extra sentence which you **DO NOT** need to use.
- Mark the corresponding letter on your **answer sheet**.

Placebo Effect

The placebo effect has sometimes been defined as a physiological effect caused by the placebo, but Moerman and Jonas have pointed out that this seems illogical, as a placebo is an inert substance that does not directly cause anything. (**51**) _____ They propose that the placebo, which may be unethical, could be avoided entirely if doctors comfort and encourage their patients' health. Ernst and Resch also attempted to distinguish between the "true" and "perceived" placebo effect, as they argued that some of the effects attributed to the placebo effect could be due to other factors.

In 1985, Irving Kirsch hypothesized that placebo effects are produced by the self-fulfilling effects of response expectancies, in which the belief that one will feel different leads a person to actually feel different. According to this theory, the belief that one has received an active treatment can produce the subjective changes thought to be produced by the real treatment. Placebos can act similarly through classical conditioning, wherein a placebo and an actual stimulus are used simultaneously until the placebo is associated with the effect from the actual stimulus. (**52**) _____ Conditioning has a longer-lasting effect, and can affect earlier stages of information processing. The expectancy effect can be enhanced through factors such as the enthusiasm of the doctor, differences in size and color of placebo pills, or the use of other interventions such as injections. In one study, the response to a placebo increased from 44% to 62% when the doctor treated them with "warmth, attention, and confidence". (**53**) _____ Those that think a treatment will work display a stronger placebo effect than those do not, as evidenced by a study of acupuncture.

Because the placebo effect is based upon expectations and conditioning, the effect disappears if the patient is told that their expectations are unrealistic, or that the placebo intervention is ineffective. (**54**) _____ It has also been reported of subjects given placebos in a trial of anti-depressants, that "Once the trial was over and the patients who had been given placebos were told as such, they quickly deteriorated."

A placebo described as a muscle relaxant will cause muscle relaxation and, if described as the opposite, muscle tension. A placebo presented as a stimulant will have this effect on heart rhythm, and blood pressure, but, when administered as a depressant, the opposite effect. The perceived consumption of caffeine has been reported to cause similar effects even when decaffeinated coffee is consumed, although a 2003 study found only limited support for this. Alcohol placebos can cause intoxication and sensorimotor impairment. Perceived ergogenic aids can increase endurance, speed and weight-lifting ability, leading to the question of whether placebos should be allowed in sport competition. Placebos can help smokers quit. (**55**) _____ Interventions such as psychotherapy can have placebo effects. The effect has been observed in the transplantation of human embryonic neurons into the brains of those with advanced Parkinson's disease.

A. A conditioned pain reduction can be totally removed when its existence is explained.

B. Both conditioning and expectations play a role in placebo effect, and make different kinds of contribution.

C. Expectancy effects have been found to occur with a range of substances.

D. They occur not only during placebo analgesia but after receiving the analgesic placebo.

E. Instead they introduced the word "meaning response" for the meaning that the brain associates with the placebo, which causes a physiological placebo effect.

F. Perceived allergens that are not truly allergenic can cause allergies.

Part Five >>>>>>

 ## Questions 56—65

- Read the following passage on pharmacogenomics.
- Fill in each blank with the correct choice **A**, **B**, **C** or **D**.
- Mark the corresponding letter on your **answer sheet**.

Pharmacogenomics

The terms pharmacogenomics and pharmacogenetics are often used interchangeably to describe a field of research focused on how genes affect individual responses to medicines. Whether a medicine works well for you or whether it causes serious side effects depends, to a certain extent, on your genes.

Just as genes contribute to whether you will be tall or short, black-haired or blond, your genes also (**56**) _____ how you will respond to medicines. Genes are like recipes and they carry instructions for making protein molecules. As medicines travel through your body, they (**57**) _____ with thousands of proteins. Small differences in the composition or quantities of these molecules can affect how medicines do their jobs.

These differences can be due to diet, level of activity, or the medicines a person takes, but they can also be due to differences in genes. By understanding the genetic basis of drug responses, scientists hope to enable doctors to (**58**) _____ the drugs and doses best suited for each individual.

While standard doses of most medicines work well for most people, some medicines don't work at all in certain people or cause annoying and sometimes dangerous side effects. For example, codeine is useless as a painkiller in nearly 10 percent of people, and an anticancer drug, 6-mercaptopurine, is extremely (**59**) _____ in a small fraction of the population.

Many pharmacogenomic findings are based on knowledge of biochemical pathways within cells. For example, scientists already knew a lot about the enzymes that break down the anticancer drug irinotecan when its toxic effects in certain patients came to light. This knowledge allowed researchers to rapidly pinpoint a genetic variant of one of these enzymes (**60**) _____ the cause of the dangerous reaction. Scientists have developed a genetic test for this variant so that doctors can adjust the dosage for those at risk for serious side effects.

Advances can also come from studies that accompany clinical drug trials. (**61**) _____ obtaining permission from participants, some pharmaceutical companies collect DNA samples from people in clinical trials. Scientists then analyze the samples together with results of the clinical trial to identify genetic variations that correlate with a drug's effectiveness or toxicity.

Pharmacogenomic researchers have already identified many genes whose variations affect drug responses. They also know where to look for the numerous others they are **(62)** _____ to discover in the future. The availability of the human genome sequence, **(63)** _____ was completed in 2003, led to the HapMap project, an international effort to catalog common genetic differences among human beings. These resources are providing a treasure trove of genetic information that is expected to speed advances in pharmacogenetics.

In the future, pharmacogenomics will **(64)** _____ enable doctors to prescribe the right dose of the right medicine the first time for everyone. This would mean that patients will receive medicines that are safer and more effective, leading to better health care overall.

Also, if scientists could identify the genetic basis for certain toxic side effects, drugs could be prescribed only to those who are not genetically at risk for these effects. This could maintain the availability of **(65)** _____ lifesaving medications that might otherwise be taken off the market.

56. A. predict   **B.** diagnose   **C.** calculate   **D.** determine

57. A. contact   **B.** connect   **C.** interact   **D.** act

58. A. prescribe   **B.** deliberate   **C.** describe   **D.** banner

59. A. toxic   **B.** effective   **C.** beneficial   **D.** fierce

60. A. with   **B.** as   **C.** for   **D.** on

61. A. Prefer   **B.** Due to   **C.** Before   **D.** After

62. A. come   **B.** bound   **C.** ready   **D.** account

63. A. where   **B.** that   **C.** which   **D.** one

64. A. seriously   **B.** therapeutically   **C.** increasingly   **D.** exclusively

65. A. frequently   **B.** consequently   **C.** infrequently   **D.** undoubtedly

Ⅲ Writing

 Question 66

- Write an essay of about 150 words on the topic "Should Nurses Go Abroad to Work?". You should base your essay on the clues given below.
- Please write your essay on the **answer sheet**.

Should Nurses Go Abroad to Work?

1. 现在很多护士想出国工作。
2. 她们选择出国工作的原因。
3. 谈谈你的想法。

医护英语水平考试(三级)

模拟训练(三)

Medical English Test System (METS)
Level 3

Ⅰ Listening

Part One >>>>>>

 ## Questions 1—5

- You will hear five extracts from conversations taking place in different clinical departments.
- Choose which case each doctor is discussing from the list **A—F**.
- Use each letter **A—F** only once. There is one extra letter which you **DO NOT** need to use.
- Mark the corresponding letter on your **answer sheet**.
- You will hear each extract twice.

Doctor 1		1
Doctor 2		2
Doctor 3		3
Doctor 4		4
Doctor 5		5

A. The patient had a history of dysuria, weight loss, night sweats and tiredness.

B. The patient received a mitral valve replacement three years ago.

C. The patient complained of fatigue, malaise, weight gain, constipation and hair loss.

D. The patient was diagnosed as having malaria after he returned from Africa.

E. The man had swollen tonsils with no exudates.

F. The rapid streptococcal antigen test of the patient is positive.

Part Two >>>>>>

 ## Questions 6—13

- You will hear a conversation between a chief physician and a patient.
- For each of the following statements, decide whether it is **True (A)** or **False (B)**. If there is not enough information to answer **True (A)** or **False (B)**, choose **Not Given (C)**.
- Mark the corresponding letter on your **answer sheet**.
- You will hear the recording twice.

---

6. The patient had a persistent pain in his abdomen, as well as the chest, back and thigh.
    A. True   **B.** False   **C.** Not Given

7. The patient received an operation for the pain 14 years ago.
    A. True   **B.** False   **C.** Not Given

8. At the beginning, the pain covered a wide range and mainly appeared on exertion.
    A. True   **B.** False   **C.** Not Given

9. In recent years, the pain intensified and the patient can hardly turn around.
    A. True   **B.** False   **C.** Not Given

10. The patient often has a feeling of fullness with a poor appetite.
    A. True   **B.** False   **C.** Not Given

11. The patient has visited the doctor for several times, but the condition was not improved.
    A. True   **B.** False   **C.** Not Given

12. The patient complained of fatigue, weakness, constipation, nocturia and cough.
    A. True   **B.** False   **C.** Not Given

13. Four days ago, the patient was admitted to the emergency room in a confused state.
    A. True   **B.** False   **C.** Not Given

Part Three >>>>>>

 ## Questions 14—20

- You will hear a conversation between the patient Krista and the nurse Shirley about her concerns on Cesarean section.
- For questions **14—20**, choose the most appropriate answer.
- Mark the corresponding letter on your **answer sheet**.
- You will hear the conversation twice.

---

14. When will Krista have a Cesarean section?
    A. Eight am this Friday.
    B. Three pm next Monday.
    C. Nine am next Monday.

15. What kind of anesthesia will Krista have for her scheduled C-section?
    A. General anesthesia.
    B. Epidural anesthesia.
    C. Spinal anesthesia.

16. What is Krista's conscious state during the C-section?
    A. She is semiconscious.
    B. She is in deep sleep.
    C. She is awake and alert.

17. What is the primary role of Krista's husband in the operating room?
    A. To provide support for Krista.
    B. To observe the process of the operation.
    C. To hold the baby.

18. Where will the patient be sent to right after the C-section?
    A. The general ward.
    B. The post anesthesia care unit.
    C. The delivery suite.

19. Which unit will the patient be transferred to when she is signed off by the anesthesiologist?
    A. The postpartum unit.
    B. The intensive care unit.
    C. The neonatal intensive care unit.

20. Which of the following about breastfeeding is NOT correct?

A. The mother can't breastfeed the baby right after the surgery because she doesn't have any milk yet.

B. Breastfeeding is encouraged for every healthy mother no matter she receives a C-section or not.

C. Breastfeeding is good for the recovery of the uterus.

Part Four >>>>>>

 ## Questions 21—25

- You will hear a talk of case history about a patient Mr. Zhang.
- Complete the notes. In each blank, write only one word.
- Write the answers on your **answer sheet**.
- You will hear the talk twice.

Case history	
Name: Zhang Hang Age: 45 Nationality: Chinese Canadian	
Present illness	Presented on September 14, 2017 with lethargy and polyuria. His family physicians noted a high serum calcium and a low serum (**21**) _____.
Past history	Undergone an emergency portacaval shunt for bleeding esophageal (**22**) _____ 20 years ago. Received one blood transfusion.
Physical examination	Fit looking with considerable anxiety. Abdominal ultrasound examination revealed a (**23**) _____ lesion in the right lobe of the liver. Soft abdomen with no organomegaly or ascites. Dynamic CT scan showed a middle solid (**24**) _____ lesion in right lobe of the liver. Doppler ultrasound of the liver vessels confirmed a portacaval shunt.
Initial treatment	Intravenous rehydration and (**25**) _____.

II Reading

Part One >>>>>

 Questions 26—35

- Read the following passage about sleep.

Sleep: A Dynamic Activity

1 Until the 1950s, most people thought of sleep as a passive, dormant part of our daily lives. We now know that our brains are very active during sleep. Moreover, sleep affects our daily functioning and our physical and mental health in many ways that we are just beginning to understand.

2 Nerve-signaling chemicals called neurotransmitters control whether we are asleep or awake by acting on different groups of nerve cells, or neurons, in the brain. Neurons in the brainstem, which connect the brain with the spinal cord, produce neurotransmitters such as serotonin and norepinephrine that keep some parts of the brain active while we are awake. Other neurons at the base of the brain begin signaling when we fall asleep. These neurons appear to "switch off" the signals that keep us awake. Research also suggests that a chemical called adenosine builds up in our blood while we are awake and causes drowsiness. This chemical gradually breaks down while we sleep.

3 During sleep, we usually pass through five phases of sleep: stages 1, 2, 3, 4, and REM (rapid eye movement) sleep. These stages progress in a cycle from stage 1 to REM sleep, then the cycle starts over again with stage 1. We spend almost 50 percent of our total sleep time in stage 2 sleep, about 20 percent in REM sleep, and the remaining 30 percent in the other stages. Infants, by contrast, spend about half of their sleep time in REM sleep.

4 During stage 1, which is light sleep, we drift in and out of sleep and can be awakened easily. Our eyes move very slowly and muscle activity slows. People awakened from stage 1 sleep often remember fragmented visual images. Many also experience sudden muscle contractions called hypnic myoclonia, often preceded by a sensation of starting to fall. These sudden movements are similar to the "jump" we make when startled. When we enter stage 2 sleep, our eye movements stop and our brain waves (fluctuations of electrical activity that can be measured by electrodes) become slower, with occasional bursts of rapid waves called sleep spindles. In stage 3, extremely slow brain waves called delta waves begin to appear, interspersed with smaller, faster waves. By stage 4, the brain produces delta waves almost exclusively. It is very difficult to wake someone during stages 3 and 4, which together are called deep sleep. There is no eye movement or muscle activity. People awakened during deep sleep do not adjust immediately and often feel groggy and disoriented for several minutes after they wake up. Some children experience bedwetting, night terrors, or sleepwalking during deep sleep.

5 When we switch into REM sleep, our breathing becomes more rapid, irregular, and shallow, our eyes jerk rapidly in various directions, and our limb muscles become temporarily paralyzed. Our heart rate increases, our blood pressure rises, and males develop penile erections. When people are awakened during REM sleep, they often describe bizarre and illogical tales—dreams.

 Questions 26—30

- Choose the most appropriate subheading from the list **A—F** for each paragraph.
- Use each letter **A—F** only once. There is one extra letter which you **DO NOT** need to use.
- Mark the corresponding letter on your **answer sheet**.

26. Paragraph 1 _____

27. Paragraph 2 _____

28. Paragraph 3 _____

29. Paragraph 4 _____

30. Paragraph 5 _____

> **A.** Body conditions during the first four stages
> **B.** Too much beyond what we know about sleep
> **C.** How much sleep do we need?
> **D.** Neurons and chemicals involved in sleep
> **E.** Body reactions during REM sleep
> **F.** Five phases of sleep in human being

Questions 31—35

- Fill in each blank with the correct answer from the list **A—F**.
- Use each letter **A—F** only once. There is one extra letter which you **DO NOT** need to use.
- Mark the corresponding letter on your **answer sheet**.

31. The stages of sleep _____ from stage 1, 2, 3, and 4 to REM sleep. Then the cycle starts over again with stage 1.

32. Whether we are asleep or awake is controlled by _____ called neurotransmitters acting on different groups of neurons in the brain.

33. There are _____ and lower brain waves during 50% of total sleep time in adults.

34. Children may experience bedwetting, night terrors or sleepwalking _____.

35. Dreams often occur _____ rather than deep sleep.

> **A.** nerve-signaling chemicals
> **B.** during deep sleep
> **C.** growing numbers
> **D.** progress in a cycle
> **E.** during REM sleep
> **F.** no eye movements

Part Two >>>>>>

 Questions 36—42

- Read the following passage about irritable bowel syndrome.
- Choose the best answer **A, B, C** or **D**.
- Mark the corresponding letter on your **answer sheet**.

Irritable Bowel Syndrome

Irritable bowel syndrome (IBS) is a common intestinal condition characterized by abdominal pain and cramps, changes in bowel movements (diarrhea, constipation, or both), gassiness, bloating, nausea, and other symptoms. There is no cure for IBS. Much about the condition remains unknown or poorly understood; however, dietary changes, drugs, and psychological treatment are often able to eliminate or substantially reduce its symptoms.

IBS was once called—among other things—colitis, spastic colon, nervous colon, and spastic bowel. Some of these names reflected the now outdated belief that IBS is a purely psychological disorder, a product of the patient's imagination. Although modern medicine recognizes that stress can trigger IBS attacks, medical specialists agree that IBS is a genuine physical disorder—or group of disorders—with specific identifiable characteristics.

Researchers remain unsure about the cause or causes of IBS. It is called a functional disorder because it is thought to result from changes in the activity of the major part of the large intestine (the colon). After food is digested by the stomach and small intestine, the undigested material passes in liquid form into the colon, which absorbs water and salts. This process may take several days. In a healthy person the colon is quiet during most of that period except after meals, when its muscles contract in a series of wavelike movements called peristalsis. Peristalsis helps absorption by bringing the undigested material into contact with the colon wall. It also pushes undigested material that has been converted into solid or semisolid feces toward the rectum, where it remains until defecation. In IBS, however, the normal rhythm and intensity of peristalsis is disrupted. Sometimes there is too little peristalsis, which can slow the passage of undigested material through the colon and cause constipation. Sometimes there is too much, which has the opposite effect and causes diarrhea.

Some kinds of food and drink appear to play a key role in triggering IBS attacks. Food and drink that healthy people can ingest without any trouble may disrupt peristalsis in IBS patients, which probably explains why IBS attacks often occur shortly after meals. Chocolate, milk products, caffeine (in coffee, tea, colas, and other drinks), and large quantities of alcohol are some of the chief culprits. Other kinds of food have also been identified as problems, however, and the pattern of what can and cannot be tolerated is different for each person. Characteristically, IBS symptoms rarely occur at night and disrupt the patient's sleep.

Stress is an important factor in IBS because of the close nervous system connections between the brain and the intestines. Although researchers do not yet understand all of the links between changes in the nervous system and IBS, they point out the similarities between mild digestive upsets and IBS. Just as healthy people can feel nauseated or have an upset stomach when under stress, people with IBS react the same way, but to a greater degree. Finally, IBS symptoms sometimes intensify during menstruation, which suggests that female reproductive hormones are another trigger.

---

36. What do the changes in bowel movements refer to in IBS?

A. Diarrhea.

B. Constipation.

C. Diarrhea alternating with constipation.

D. All of above.

37. Which one of the names apparently reflected that IBS was a purely psychological disorder?

A. Colitis.　　　　　　　　　B. Spastic colon.

C. Nervous colon.　　　　　　D. Spastic bowel.

38. Why is IBS called a functional disorder according to the passage?

A. The function of the large intestine may be disturbed.

B. There are some morphologic abnormalities in the large intestine.

C. It is thought to result from structural changes of the colon.

D. Researchers do not know the causes of IBS.

39. In IBS constipation may occur when _____.

A. normal treatment is disrupted

B. the rhythm and intensity of peristalsis is too little

C. a patient has diet with too much fiber and lower fat

D. stress is removed

40. What may be the meaning of the word "culprits" in the fourth paragraph?

A. Mediators.　　　　　　　　B. Therapeutic agents.

C. Pathogenic factors.　　　　D. Nerve transmitters.

41. Which one of the following factors does NOT contribute to the IBS?

A. Stress.　　　　　　　　　　B. Hormones.

C. Food and drink.　　　　　　D. Mild digestive upsets.

42. Which of the following statements is true about IBS?

A. The symptoms of IBS are growing steadily worse over time.

B. IBS is a purely psychological disorder rather than a physical disorder.

C. There is abnormal rhythm and intensity of peristalsis in IBS.

D. Attacks of IBS usually disrupt the patient's sleep at night.

Part Three　>>>>>>

Questions 43—50

• Read the following passage about new weapon to fight cancer.

- For each of the following statements, decide whether it is **True (A)** or **False (B)**. If there is not enough information to answer **True (A)** or **False (B)**, choose **Not Given (C)**.
- Mark the corresponding letter on your **answer sheet**.

New Weapon to Fight Cancer

British scientists are preparing to launch trials of a radical new way to fight cancer, which kills tumors by infecting them with viruses like the common cold.

If successful, virus therapy could eventually form a third pillar alongside radiotherapy and chemotherapy in the standard arsenal against cancer, while avoiding some of the debilitating side-effects.

Leonard Seymour, a professor of gene therapy at Oxford University, who has been working on the virus therapy with colleagues in London and the US, will lead the trials later this year. Cancer Research UK said yesterday that it was exciting by the potential of Prof Seymour's pioneering techniques.

One of the country's leading geneticists, Prof Seymour has been working with viruses that kill cancer cells directly, while avoiding harm to healthy tissue. "In principle, you've got something which could be many times more effective than regular chemotherapy," he said.

Cancer-killing viruses exploit the fact that cancer cells suppress the body's local immune system. "If a cancer doesn't do that, the immune system wipes it out. If you can get a virus into a tumor, viruses find them a very good place to be because there's no immune system to stop them replicating. You can regard it as the cancer's Achilles' heel."

Only a small amount of the virus needs to get to the cancer. "They replicate, they get a million copies in each cell and the cell bursts and they infect the tumor cells adjacent and repeat the process," said Prof Seymour.

Preliminary research on mice shows that the viruses work well on tumors resistant to standard cancer drugs. "It's an interesting possibility that they may have an advantage in killing drug-resistant tumors, which could be quite different to anything we've had before."

Researchers have known for some time that viruses can kill tumor cells and some aspects of the work have already been published in scientific journals. American scientists have previously injected viruses directly into tumors but this technique will not work if the cancer is inaccessible or has spread throughout the body.

Prof Seymour's innovative solution is to mask the virus from the body's immune system, effectively allowing the viruses to do what chemotherapy drugs do—spread through the blood and reach tumors wherever they are. The big hurdle has always been to find a way to deliver viruses to tumors via the bloodstream without the body's immune system destroying them on the way.

"What we've done is making chemical modifications to the virus to put a polymer coat around it—it's a stealth virus when you inject it," he said.

After the stealth virus infects the tumor, it replicates, but the copies do not have the chemical modifications. If they escape from the tumor, the copies will be quickly recognized and mopped up by the body's immune system.

The therapy would be especially useful for secondary cancers, called metastases, which sometimes spread around the body after the first tumor appears. "There's an awful statistic of patients in the west ... with malignant cancers; 75% of them go on to die from metastases," said Prof Seymour.

43. Virus therapy, if successful, has an advantage in eliminating side-effects.

    A. True   **B.** False   **C.** Not Given

44. Cancer Research UK is quite hopeful about Professor Seymour's work on the virus therapy.

    A. True   **B.** False   **C.** Not Given

45. Virus can kill cancer cells and stop them from growing again.

    A. True   **B.** False   **C.** Not Given

46. Cancer's Achilles' heel refers to the fact that virus may stay safely in a tumor and replicate.

    A. True   **B.** False   **C.** Not Given

47. To infect the cancer cells, a good deal of viruses should be injected into the tumor.

    A. True   **B.** False   **C.** Not Given

48. Researches on animals indicate that virus could be used as a new way to treat drug-resistant tumors.

    A. True   **B.** False   **C.** Not Given

49. Uncoated adenovirus and vaccinia are likely to be examined in the first clinical trials.

    A. True   **B.** False   **C.** Not Given

50. The chemical modifications to the virus are Prof Seymour's innovative solution.

    A. True   **B.** False   **C.** Not Given

Part Four >>>>>>

 ## Questions 51—55

- Read the following passage about tickling and laughter. Five sentences have been removed from the passage.
- Fill in each blank with the most appropriate sentence from the list **A—F**. There is one extra sentence which you **DO NOT** need to use.
- For each space (**51—55**), mark one letter **A—F** on your **answer sheet**.

Tickling and Laughter

The fingers of an outstretched arm are nearing your body; you bend away folding your torso, bending your head to your shoulder in hopes that you don't get tickled; but the inevitable occurs as what you anticipated—you are tickled and in hysterics you chuckle, titter, and burst into uncontrollable laughter. (**51**) _____.

Tickling is caused by a light sensation across our skin. At times the light sensation can cause itching; however, most of the time the light touch causes giggling. If a feather is gently moved across the surface of the skin, this can also cause tickling and giggling. Heavy laughter is caused by someone or something placing repeated pressure on a person and tickling a particular area. (**52**) _____ Yngve Zotterman from Karolinksk Institute has found that tickling sensations involve signals from nerve fibers. These nerve fibers are associated with pain and touch. Also, Zotterman discovered tickling sensations to be associated with sense of touch but not just with nerve fibers because people who have lost pain sensations still laugh when tickled.

(**53**) _____ Laughter requires the coordination of many muscles throughout the body. Laughter also increases blood pressure and heart rate, changes breathing, reduces levels of certain neurochemicals (catecholamines, hormones) and provides a boost to the immune system. Can laughter improve health? It may be a good way for people to relax since muscle tension is reduced after laughing. Human tests have found some evidence that humorous videos and tapes can reduce feelings of pain, prevent negative stress reactions and boost the brain's biological battle against infection.

(**54**) _____ In one new study, researchers used imaging equipment to photograph the brain activity of healthy volunteers while they underwent a sidesplitting assignment of reading written jokes, viewing cartoons from *The New Yorker* magazine as well as "The

Far Side" and listening to digital recordings of laughter. Preliminary results indicate that the humor-processing pathway includes parts of the frontal lobe brain area, important for cognitive processing; the supplementary motor area, important for movement; and the nucleus accumbens, associated with pleasure. Investigations support the notion that parts of the frontal lobe are involved in humor. Subjects' brains were imaged while they listened to jokes. **(55)** _____ A study also compared healthy individuals with people who had damage to their frontal lobes, and the subjects with the damaged frontal lobes were more likely to choose a wrong punch line to written jokes and didn't laugh or smile as much at funny cartoons or jokes.

A. Why do we laugh when we are tickled?

B. Researchers believe we process humor and laughter through a complex pathway of brain activity that encompasses three main brain components.

C. The sites tickled often are feet, toes, sides, underarms, and neck which cause a great deal of laughter.

D. The brain's "funny bone" is located at the right frontal lobe just above the right eye and appears critical to our ability to recognize a joke.

E. Research has shown that laughing is more than just a person's voice and movement.

F. An area of the frontal lobe was activated only when they thought a joke was funny.

Part Five >>>>>>

 Question 56—65

- Read the following passage about magnet therapy.
- Fill in each blank with the correct choice **A**, **B**, **C** or **D**.
- Mark the corresponding letter on your **answer sheet**.

Magnet Therapy

Magnet therapy, which is a $5-billion market worldwide, is a form of alternative medicine which claims that magnetic fields have healing powers. Magnetic devices that are claimed to be **(56)** _____ include magnetic bracelets, insoles, wrist and knee bands, back and neck braces, and even pillows and mattresses. Their annual sales are estimated at $300m in the United States and more than a billion dollars globally. They have been **(57)** _____ to cure a vast array of ills, particularly pain.

The therapy works on the (**58**) _____ of balancing electrical energy in the body by pulsating magnetic waves through different parts of the body. The electrical currents generated by magnets increase the blood flow and oxygen which helps to heal many of the ailments and countless numbers of people around the world are using magnets and this therapy is usually prescribed to relieve pain—(**59**) _____ muscle and joint pains, but occasionally headache, carpal tunnel syndrome and other types of pains as well. (**60**) _____ its many applications are strains, sprains of the spine, neck or limbs, hip and joint pain, arthritis and chronic pelvic pain, plus healing of bone fractures and some proponents even advocate magnets to relieve stress, combat infections and prevent seizures.

The practice of magnetic therapy as an alternative medication has led to the growth of an entire industry though there is no concrete evidence on the working and the effectiveness of this type of therapy. Still those who practice it, strongly believe that certain ailments can be treated if the patient is (**61**) _____ to magnetic fields but at the same time there is a strong resentment from the medical establishment and critics claim that most magnets don't have the strength to effect the various organs and tissues within the body and it is a product of Pseudoscience and is not based on proper research and analysis. There are few reported complications of magnetic therapy and the World Health Organization says (**62**) _____ levels of magnetic energy is not harmful. Documented side effects are not life-threatening and include pain, nausea and dizziness that disappeared when the magnets were removed. It is also advised that pregnant women should not get magnetic therapy treatments. Those with pacemakers should avoid magnetic devices as well as those who are taking an MRI or radiology treatment, (**63**) _____ the magnetic forces can disrupt the equipment used during those procedures.

Researchers at Baylor University Medical Center recently conducted a double-blind study (**64**) _____ the use of concentric-circle magnets to relieve chronic pain in 50 post-polio patients. Active as well as placebo magnets ranging from 300—500 gauss were placed on the affected area of each patient for 45 minutes. A (**65**) _____ number of patients (76 percent) reported less pain when using the active magnets as opposed to those who reported less pain while using a placebo magnet (19 percent).

Magnet therapy is gaining popularity; however, the scientific evidence to support the success of this therapy is lacking. More scientifically sound studies are needed in order to fully understand the effects that magnets can have on the body and the possible benefits or dangers that could result from their use.

56. A. therapeutic   **B.** diagnostic   **C.** stimulative   **D.** aggressive

57. A. recommended   **B.** advertised   **C.** noted   **D.** installed

58. **A.** therapy   **B.** remedy   **C.** principle   **D.** dosage

59. **A.** effectively   **B.** fortunately   **C.** virtually   **D.** primarily

60. **A.** With   **B.** Through   **C.** Among   **D.** Between

61. **A.** evolved   **B.** exposed   **C.** involved   **D.** proposed

62. **A.** low   **B.** minimal   **C.** fewer   **D.** less

63. **A.** by   **B.** as   **C.** in   **D.** owning

64. **A.** in   **B.** up   **C.** on   **D.** as

65. **A.** irrational   **B.** equivalent   **C.** experimental   **D.** significant

Ⅲ Writing

 Question 66

- Write an essay of about 150 words on the topic "Should Induced Abortion Be Controlled?" You should base your essay on the clues given below.
- Please write your essay on the **answer sheet**.

Should Induced Abortion Be Controlled?

1. 人工流产会影响女性健康
2. 人工流产是不人道的
3. 因此,……

医护英语水平考试(三级)

模拟训练(四)

Medical English Test System (METS)
Level 3

I　Listening

Part One　>>>>>>

 ## Questions 1—5

- You will hear five extracts from conversations taking place in different clinical departments.
- Choose which case each doctor is discussing from the list **A—F**.
- Use each letter **A—F** only once. There is one extra letter which you **DO NOT** need to use.
- Mark the corresponding letter on your **answer sheet**.
- You will hear each extract twice.

Doctor 1	1
Doctor 2	2
Doctor 3	3
Doctor 4	4
Doctor 5	5

A. The patient has a high risk of having cardiovascular disease.

B. The patient feels some discomfort after the treatment of ovarian carcinoma.

C. The patient has myelofibrosis and will receive treatment.

D. The patient has intertrochanteric fracture.

E. The patient has severe depression.

F. The patient is going to have surgery.

Part Two >>>>>

 Questions 6—13

- You will hear a conversation between a reporter and a WHO official.
- For each of the following statements, decide whether it is **True (A)** or **False (B)**. If there is not enough information to answer **True (A)** or **False (B)**, choose **Not Given (C)**.
- Mark the corresponding letter on your **answer sheet**.
- You will hear the recording twice.

---

6. About 90% of all deaths worldwide are caused by NCDs.
   A. True   **B.** False   **C.** Not Given

7. People who died prematurely usually died before reaching 70 years of age.
   A. True   **B.** False   **C.** Not Given

8. Tobacco use is one of the top reasons for premature death.
   A. True   **B.** False   **C.** Not Given

9. Prevention and control of NCDs is imperative for the 21st century.
   A. True   **B.** False   **C.** Not Given

10. Most NCD deaths occur in low- and middle-income countries.
    A. True   **B.** False   **C.** Not Given

11. Six African countries have failed to make any progress against such deaths.
    A. True   **B.** False   **C.** Not Given

12. WHO's mission is to provide leadership and the evidence base for international action on surveillance, prevention and control of NCDs.
    A. True   **B.** False   **C.** Not Given

13. A global dialogue to address the critical gap in financing for national NCD responses was held early this month.
    A. True   **B.** False   **C.** Not Given

Part Three >>>>>

 Questions 14—20

- You will hear a discussion among an instructor and two medical students.
- For questions **14—20**, choose the most appropriate answer.

- Mark the corresponding letter on your **answer sheet**.
- You will hear the discussion twice.

---

14. Double pneumonia is an infection of _____.

    A. both lungs   **B.** both kidneys   **C.** both eyes

15. Double pneumonia may be caused by the following EXCEPT _____.

    A. bacteria   **B.** virus   **C.** pollutants

16. Symptoms of pneumonia include the following EXCEPT _____.

    A. a high fever, chills, or shaking

    B. coughing up thick mucus or phlegm

    C. stomach pain when coughing or breathing

17. What are the complications of pneumonia?

    A. Spesis and tuberculosis.

    B. Spesis and lung abscesses.

    C. Tuberculosis and abscesses.

18. The pleurae are two membranes that line the outside of the lungs within the _____.

    A. chest cavity   **B.** oral cavity   **C.** abdominal cavity

19. Patients who have bacterial pneumonia will need _____.

    A. antibiotic therapy

    B. intravenous antimicrobial therapy

    C. hydrotherapy

20. Which of the following statements about coughing is WRONG?

    A. Coughing can be unpleasant.

    B. Coughing helps the body rid itself of the infection.

    C. People who have double pneumonia should take a cough suppressant medicine.

Part Four >>>>>>

Questions 21—25

- You will hear a speech on smoking e-cigarettes, or vaping.
- Complete the notes. In each blank, write only one word.
- Write the answers on your **answer sheet**.
- You will hear the speech twice.

Notes:

Many people might be tempted to turn to electronic cigarettes as a way to ease the transition from traditional cigarettes to non-smoking. Here are some truth known about smoking e-cigarettes, or vaping.

- Vaping is less harmful than traditional smoking.

  Regular tobacco cigarettes contain 7,000 chemicals, many of which are (**21**) _____ .

  E-cigarettes expose you to fewer toxic chemicals than traditional cigarettes.

- Vaping is still bad for health because nicotine is still the primary (**22**) _____ in both regular cigarettes and e-cigarettes.

  Nicotine is a toxic substance which may increase the heart rate and the likelihood of having a heart attack indirectly.

  There are many unknowns about vaping.

- Electronic cigarettes are just as addictive as traditional ones.

  E-cigarette users may get even more nicotine because they can buy extra-strength cartridges, which have a higher (**23**) _____ of nicotine.

- E-cigarettes have not received Food and Drug Administration approval as smoking (**24**) _____ devices.

- E-cigarettes are more (**25**) _____ among youth than any traditional tobacco products.

Ⅱ Reading

Part One >>>>>

 Questions 26—35

- Read the following passage about diet and pregnancy.

Women Who Eat Less Fruit and More Fast Food Take Longer to Get Pregnant

1 Women may be harming their chances of getting pregnant because they're avoiding fruit, or eating too much junk food, a study has found. Australian researchers found that women who ate fewer than three pieces of fruit a month took 50 percent longer to conceive than women who ate fruit three or more times a month. Women who eat less fruit and more fast food take longer to get pregnant and are less likely to conceive within a year, according to a study by researchers at the University of Adelaide's Robinson Research Institute.

2 Junk food consumption was also analyzed, and women who rarely ate fast food got pregnant a month quicker, on average than women who ate fast food four times a week or more. While the intake of fruit and fast food affected the time it took to get pregnant, the researchers found intake of green leafy vegetables or fish did not.

3 As parents are getting older, one in six couples trying to conceive now struggle to get pregnant and keeping a healthy weight and diet is a key way to improve chances, independent experts warned. However they added there were also many myths about fertility, including the suggestion that fruit should be avoided. The study, which is published in the journal *Human Reproduction*, saw 5,598 women questioned about their diet during their first antenatal visit. The women, who were from the UK, Ireland, Australia and New Zealand, had not had a baby before.

4 Among all the couples in the study, 468 (8 percent) were classified as infertile (defined as taking longer than a year to conceive) and 2,204 (39 percent) conceived within a month. When researchers looked at the impact of diet on infertility, they found that in women with the lowest intake of fruit, the risk of infertility increased from 8 percent to 12 percent, and in those who ate fast food four or more times a week, the risk of infertility increased from 8 percent to 16 percent. Professor Claire Roberts, from the University of Adelaide, who led the study, said: "These findings show that eating a good quality diet that includes fruit and minimizing fast food consumption improves fertility and reduces the time it takes to get pregnant." Melanie McGrice, who was not involved with the study, said: "As a fertility dietician, I'm seeing more and more women who incorrectly think that they should be avoiding fruit in an effort to help them conceive." Compared to women who ate fruit three or more times a day in the month before conception, women who ate fruit less than one to three times a month took half a month longer to become pregnant. Similarly, compared to women who never or rarely ate fast food, women who consumed fast food four or more times a week took nearly a month longer to become pregnant.

5 This study demonstrates that fruit consumption is not only safe, but beneficial for most women to optimize their fertility. Fruit is rich in antioxidants, vitamins and phytochemicals, and should not be lumped into the same basket as sugar and soft drinks. The researchers are continuing their work and plan to identify particular dietary patterns, rather than individual food groups, that may be associated with how long it takes women to become pregnant.

Questions 26—30

- Choose the most appropriate subheading from the list **A—F** for each paragraph.
- Use each letter **A—F** only once. There is one extra letter which you **DO NOT** need

to use.

- Mark the corresponding letter on your **answer sheet**.

26. Paragraph 1 _____

27. Paragraph 2 _____

28. Paragraph 3 _____

29. Paragraph 4 _____

30. Paragraph 5 _____

A. Analysis of junk food consumption

B. Roles of fruit in improving conception

C. Food groups that may affect the chances of conception

D. Findings showing the relation between diet and fertility

E. The key way to improve chances of conception

F. Fruit acting as sugar and soft drinks

Questions 31—35

- Fill in each blank with the correct answer from the list **A—F**.
- Use each letter **A—F** only once. There is one extra letter which you **DO NOT** need to use.
- Mark the corresponding letter on your **answer sheet**.

31. A study made by researchers at the University of Adelaide's Robinson Research Institute showed that who eat less fruit and more junk food take longer to _____ and are less likely to conceive within a year.

32. _____, women who rarely ate fast food got pregnant a month quicker than women who ate fast food four times a week or more.

33. Experts added there were many _____ including the suggestion that fruit should be avoided.

34. Melaine McGrice, a _____, holds that more and more women have the wrong idea that they should be avoiding fruit in an effort to help them conceive.

35. Rich in antioxidants, vitamins and phytochemicals, fruit should not _____ the same basket as sugar and soft drinks.

A. On average

B. be classified as

C. fertility dietician(s)

D. get pregnant

E. myth(s) about fertility

F. be lumped into

Part Two $>>>>>>$

 Questions 36—42

- Read the following passage about NHS cancer screening.
- Choose the best answer **A**, **B**, **C** or **D**.
- Mark the corresponding letter on your **answer sheet**.

Nearly Half a Million Women Missed out on National Health Service Cancer Screening

Nearly half a million women missed out on NHS (National Health Service) cancer screening because of an IT error, the government has admitted, adding that hundreds may have died as a result.

Jeremy Hunt, the health and social care secretary, has apologized for the glitch which meant 450,000 women were never sent letters inviting them to routine breast cancer checkups. He admitted up to 270 of those affected could have died prematurely as a result of the error and officials told *The Independent* there may be more women whose cancer was caught at a later and less treatable stage. The government announced an independent inquiry into the full extent of what charities have called an "appalling error", and said it would begin the "distressing" process of contacting families to establish whether they are owed compensation.

The following are some fast facts of NHS cancer screening.

What is NHS breast cancer screening?

Women aged 50 to 70 are invited for an X-ray mammogram every three years to detect any lumps or abnormalities that could be or become breast cancer.

How many women are screened?

Around 2.5 million women are invited to breast screening each year. In 2016/17 just 70 percent took up screening—a record low—and 18,400 cancers were picked up.

What is the evidence for it?

The benefits of national breast screening are contested, particularly in older women. While early diagnosis helps maximize chances of survival, critics say large numbers of women are subjected to harm from X-rays, biopsies and preventative mastectomies for lumps that may never become cancer.

A technical issue dating back to 2009 and only caught in 2018 was responsible for some women in England missing out on the last of their regular invitations for screening.

In a statement today, Mr. Hunt announced the "best estimate" is that between 135 and 270 women "had their lives shortened as a result".

"I am advised that it is unlikely to be more than this range, and may be considerably less," he added.

"Tragically there are likely to be some people in this group who would be alive today had this failure not happened. "

These numbers are based on statistical estimates of the rates of cancers caught for every woman screened, however the independent review will establish exactly how many women were affected by reviewing case notes.

It will also try to determine how the issues went unnoticed for the best part of a decade.

The NHS currently screens women between the ages of 50 and 70 for breast cancer every three years, but only women aged between 68 and 71 were affected by this issue.

The glitch first came to light in January after an upgrade to the national screening IT system which found women enrolled in a long-running study, the AgeX trial, led by Oxford University, were not receiving their final screening invitation around age 70.

This led to a wider review which the problem and other issues were replicated across England.

Of the affected group, 309,000 women are believed to still be alive and will receive a letter by the end of May telling them they may have missed screening and inviting them for a checkup now.

Mr. Hunt admitted that among the women contacted there are likely to be people who have recently had a terminal cancer diagnosis and "apologized wholeheartedly" on behalf of the government, NHS England and Public Health England for the failure.

"In addition, as soon as possible we will make our best endeavor to contact the next of kin of those we believe have missed a scan and subsequently died of breast cancer," the health secretary added.

"As well as apologizing to families affected, we wish to offer any further advice they might find helpful including a process to establish whether a missed scan was a likely cause of death and compensation is therefore payable.

"We recognize this will be incredibly distressing for some families. "

Public Health England said it is not possible to estimate how many women in this group may have cancer that was picked up late, or is currently undiagnosed, until these catchup screenings are complete.

Across England, PHE invites 2.5 million women, aged 50 to 70, to breast cancer screening each year, around 70 percent attended in 2016 - 17 and 18,400 cancers were picked up.

The AgeX trial is being conducted to determine the usefulness of screening women younger than 50 and older women, up to the age of 73, as its benefits are currently disputed.

36. Why did Health and Social Health secretary Jeremy Hunt apologize?

A. Because 400,000 women were never sent letters inviting them to routine breast cancer checkups.

B. Because some women were never sent letters inviting them to routine breast cancer checkups.

C. Because 450,000 women were never sent letters inviting them to routine breast cancer checkups.

D. Because all the women were never sent letters inviting them to routine breast cancer checkups.

37. What is NHS breast cancer screening?

A. It is an X-ray examination for women between the age of 60 and 70 to detect lumps or abnormalities that could be breast cancer.

B. It is an X-ray mammogram for women between the age of 50 and 70 to detect lumps or abnormalities that could be breast cancer.

C. It is an X-ray light examination for women between the age of 40 and 70 to detect lumps or abnormalities that could be breast cancer.

D. It is an X-ray light for women between the age of 30 and 70 to detect lumps or abnormalities that could be breast cancer.

38. How many women took up breast screening in 2016?

A. Around 1.75 million women took up breast screening in 2016.

B. Around 2.50 million women took up breast screening in 2016.

C. Around 2.00 million women took up breast screening in 2016.

D. Around 1.84 million women took up breast screening in 2016.

39. Which of the following statements about the national breast screening is true?

A. The benefits of national breast screening are admitted, particularly in older women.

B. The benefits of national breast screening are applauded, particularly in older women.

C. The benefits of national breast screening are objected, particularly in older women.

D. The benefits of national breast screening are questioned, particularly in older women.

40. What does the "best estimate" mean?

A. It means that at most 270 women may have their lives shortened because of the error.

B. It means that at least 135 women may have their lives shortened because of the error.

C. It means that a large number of women have their lives shortened because of the error.

D. It means that it is still unknown that how many women have been influenced.

41. What will NHS do for women who missed out breast cancer screening?

   A. NHS will send a letter telling the women they may have missed screening.

   B. NHS will send a letter telling the women they may have missed screening and inviting them for a checkup now.

   C. NHS will send a letter telling the women they may have missed a checkup.

   D. NHS will send a letter telling the women they may have missed the optional cure time.

42. What will NOT be done for women who died of breast cancer as a result of missing out breast cancer screening?

   A. Their families may be contacted and receive apologies.

   B. Their families may be offered some helpful advice.

   C. Their families may be asked questions about their distress.

   D. Their families may receive compercations.

Part Three >>>>>>

 ## Questions 43—50

- Read the following passage about "third-hand" smoke.
- For each of the following statements, decide whether it is **True (A)** or **False (B)**. If there is not enough information to answer **True (A)** or **False (B)**, choose **Not Given (C)**.
- Mark the corresponding letter on your **answer sheet**.

" Third-hand " Smoke in Carpet and Furniture Could Pose Health Risk

Scientists have called for more research into the risk posed by "third-hand smoke" after finding chemicals from cigarette fumes account for nearly a third of the air particles in non-smoking environments.

US researchers found that potentially harmful chemicals from tobacco smoke get trapped in clothes, furniture and carpets but can become airborne again and be circulated through office blocks, schools or other nominally smoke-free buildings.

Unlike direct smoking, or passive "secondhand" smoke—being in a room or vehicle while someone is smoking—the health risks of third-hand smoke on surfaces and in the air are less well established.

Laboratory tests have shown indirect exposure with tobacco residues, commonly on skin, clothes or surfaces, can "detrimentally affect growth and immunity in mice", the authors write.

Experts said this could also be a concern for babies in the homes of smokers who are lying on furniture or carpets where these particles may have settled. Third-hand smoke is smoke that clings to carpets, furniture, clothing, and drapery, therefore contaminating them with harmful toxins and carcinogens can be acquired through first and second-hand smoke. This means that living in the same house with a smoker or spending a large amount of time around one can pose a great threat, and it can especially affect babies and toddlers, who spend a lot of time crawling and sitting on carpets and floors. In a study published in January 2009, researchers telephoned laypeople to ask whether or not they agreed with the idea that "Breathing air in a room today where people smoked yesterday can harm the health of infants and children." 65 percent of people who didn't smoke believed in the veracity of this statement, opposed to 43 percent of smokers.

The problem is caused by nicotine residue sticking to indoor surfaces, which later interacts with nitrous acid formed from the gas nitrous oxide, which is released by car exhausts and gas appliances.

When these chemicals combine, they can form tobacco-specific nitrosamines (TSNAs) which can cause cancer, previous studies have shown.

The latest results, published in the journal *Science Advances* today, warn that not only are these chemicals on surfaces, but also they can get back into the air and spread further afield.

This could also occur in electronic cigarettes, which also contain nicotine and are used in indoor public spaces much more frequently than conventional cigarettes, the authors said.

"In an empty classroom, where smoking has not been allowed in some time, we found that 29 percent of the entire indoor aerosol mass air particles contained third-hand smoke chemical species," said Dr. Anita Avery from Drexel University, Philadelphia.

"This was obviously quite startling and raised many questions about how that much third-hand smoke could be lingering in a non-smoking, ventilated room."

To investigate their findings further the researchers ran laboratory trials using sealed containers, one of which was filled with cigarette smoke, and then subsequently flushed with air from outdoors.

The following day they pumped in filtered air to mimic a draft or ventilation system and measured the particle content and found it was 13 percent higher in the air that had passed through the smoking container.

It's clear now that the public needs to be more aware of the dangers of third-hand smoking, because it poses a great threat to friends and relatives—particularly children of smokers. Before our society can be rid of smoking and its harmful effects, we need to understand all the ways in which we can be harmed by it.

43. US researchers found that potentially harmful chemicals from tobacco smoke may get trapped in clothes, furniture and carpets.

    A. True   **B.** False   **C.** Not Given

44. The toxic ingredients contained in third-hand smoke include hydrocyanic acid, butane, toluene, arsenic, lead, carbon monoxide, radioactive polonium-210 and a dozen other highly carcinogenic compounds.

    A. True   **B.** False   **C.** Not Given

45. Potentially harmful chemicals from tobacco smoke cann't become airborne again.

    A. True   **B.** False   **C.** Not Given

46. Indirect exposure with tobacco residues could be a concern for babies in the homes of smokers who are lying on furniture or carpets where these particles may have settled.

    A. True   **B.** False   **C.** Not Given

47. Nicotine reacts with nitrous oxide, which is released from car exhausts and gas appliances.

    A. True   **B.** False   **C.** Not Given

48. Third-hand smoke can have a big impact on the health of children, and it can also harm the respiratory system of adults.

    A. True   **B.** False   **C.** Not Given

49. Electronic cigarettes do not contain nicotine.

    A. True   **B.** False   **C.** Not Given

50. Laboratory trials were conducted for further study.

    A. True   **B.** False   **C.** Not Given

Part Four   >>>>>>

 ## Questions 51—55

- Read the following passage about workplace stress. Five sentences have been removed from the passage.
- Fill in each blank with the most appropriate sentence from the list **A—F**. There is one extra sentence which you **DO NOT** need to use.
- Mark the corresponding letter on your **answer sheet**.

Workplace Stress Should be Regulated as Safety Hazard

A third of people in Britain have experienced suicidal feelings, according to one of the largest ever reports on the nation's mental health and the growing toll of an unchecked stress epidemic. The report by the Mental Health Foundation (MHF) calls for societal change in the way mental health is treated, alongside new rules for employers to treat stress and mental health risks as seriously as physical health and safety. Launched to coincide with *Mental Health Awareness Week*, "The Stress: Are We Coping?" Report is thought to be the most comprehensive look at the damage being caused by self-neglect. Figures released today from a survey of more than 4,600 UK adults found three out of four have felt overwhelmed or are unable to cope in the past year because of stress—though this was 81 percent among women. **(51)** _____

Thirty-two percent of adults said they had experienced suicidal feelings as a result of stress, while 16 percent of adults said they had self-harmed as a result of stress with women and younger adults most likely to be affected. **(52)** _____ To address this crisis the MHF is calling on the government to introduce new standards for employers, to consider psychological hazards in workplace safety assessments. "There are very few workplaces left in the UK in which employees working with hazardous chemicals would not be provided with protective equipment, and failures resulting in injury or even death prosecuted," the report says.

"We do not currently adopt the same attitudes and behaviors towards psychological hazards." These hazards are any mental health stressors which overwhelm coping mechanisms which include taking breaks and leaving on time and ability to work safely, and breaches should be enforced, the MHF says. It also calls for a "minimum of two mental health days" for nurses, teachers, police officers and other public sector staff working twice as hard in the face of budget cuts and staff shortages. **(53)** _____

"Introducing and incentivizing the use of mental health days could help to prevent stress escalating and turning into longer-term sickness absence by encouraging self-care," the report says. "Stress is one of the great public health challenges of our time, but it still isn't being taken as seriously as physical health concerns," said MHF director Isabella Goldie.

(54) _____ It is also linked to physical health problems like heart disease, problems with our immune system, insomnia and digestive problems. There needs to be equitable access to specialist support and awareness of how stress impacts us and how it can be addressed. "We also need to change at a societal level," Ms. Goldie said. "This includes ensuring that employers treat stress and mental health problems as seriously as physical safety." Catherine Gamble, professional lead for Mental Health at the Royal College of Nursing, said: "Stress isn't a mental illness in itself, but all mental health nurses know that we are all vulnerable to it and that if left unmanaged, stress can be a precursor to more serious health conditions.

"What's striking is the amount of clinical evidence we have nowadays about the physical impact of stress—we now know it leads to an increased risk of heart disease, insomnia and damage to our immune systems." A Department of Health and Social Care spokesperson said: "Tackling stress through positive mental health support not only improves our lives as individuals, but makes good business sense—failure to adequately support the workforce is costing our economy up to £99bn per year.

"In their roles as employers the civil service and NHS are adopting new standards around mental health, as set out in the recent independent review into mental health in the workplace commissioned by the prime minister. (**55**) _____ "

A. It comes the week after Glasgow University research found that one in nine people between the ages of 18 and 34 in Scotland had attempted suicide.

B. Workplace stress should be regulated as safety hazard because one third of Britons admit feeling suicidal.

C. This includes implementing mental health plans at work, developing awareness, and monitoring health and wellbeing.

D. Stress and mental health is the fourth most common reason for workplace absence, but half of workers make up another excuse when they feel too stressed to come to work.

E. This is a sign of pressures going beyond the stresses of everyday life which can lead to more serious mental health problems, and the MHF report found evidence of this.

F. It is a significant factor in mental health problems including anxiety and depression.

Part Five >>>>>>

 ## Questions 56—65

- Read the following passage about genes and skin tans.
- Fill in each blank with the correct choice **A, B, C** or **D.**
- Mark the corresponding letter on your **answer sheet**.

Genes Controlling Whether Skin Tans or Burns Discovered by Scientists

Largest study of its kind helps scientists understand genetic basis for skin cancer. Sections of DNA that appear to play a role in controlling whether an individual's skin burns or tans have been located by scientists. In the largest genetic study of its kind, which used data from nearly 200,000 people, they (**56**) _____ the groundwork for genetic tests that could predict people's responses to sunlight. It is thought the discovery could also help researchers understand the onset of skin cancer—which (**57**) _____ 150,000 new patients in the UK every year.

Lead author of the study Dr. Mario Falchi, a researcher at King's College London, told *The Independent* that "a good percentage" of the sunburn genes which were identified also involved in skin cancer. It is a common knowledge that sunburn is a major risk factor in the development of skin cancer. Understanding the genetics of tanning therefore also means understanding the genetics of this condition, which is the most common type of cancer in people of European descent. Dr. Falchi said their work also helped explain the phenomenon familiar to many of the friend with a similar complexion who turns a different color when catching some rays.

Darker-skinned people are (**58**) _____ more resistant to the harmful effects of sunlight, but the scientists' work suggested there are genetic factors besides natural skin colour that can (**59**) _____ people from the sun. "Some of these genes involved in skin cancer probably have nothing to do with pigmentation," he said. "This may explain why for example the person next to you in the park gets completely red, while you get tanned, and you have exactly the same skin colour. There is (**60**) _____ for people with the same pigmentation."

The research was (**61**) _____ using an enormous quantity of genetic data taken from the UK Biobank, which contains information about people's health and wellbeing that can be used by researchers. Through this resource, Dr. Falchi and his colleagues had access to genetic information (**62**) _____ tens of thousands of people of European ancestry who had self-reported on their tendency to tan or burn.

This information ranged from those who said they always burned and never tanned to those who tanned without burning. The scientists then explored the genetic variability between all of these people, and ultimately pinpointed 10 new genetic regions that appeared to be linked with tanning. Their results were published in the journal *Nature Communications*.

This discovery confirmed previous work (**63**) _____ the genetic underpinnings of tanning and sunburn, and doubled the number of regions known to be involved.

"By using a very large sample size we are able to identify almost all the genes involved in determining a particularly trait—which is very interesting because once this can be defined you can develop some real genetic prediction tests," said Dr. Falchi.

However, he noted that the problem of sunburn is easy to (**64**) _____ without genetic tests, as it is essentially an issue of behavior change. "Getting tanned is a trend that started in the 1920—before no one wanted to be tanned and they wanted to be as white as possible," he noted.

The history of tanning itself can be traced back to the fashion designer Coco Chanel, who accidentally became sunburned when on holiday and unintentionally sparked a new trend that has continued to this day.

According to Cancer Research UK, almost nine out of 10 cases of melanoma—the most serious form of skin cancer—could be (**65**) _____ by "enjoying the sun safely and avoiding using sunbeds". Dr. Falchi said that regardless of genetics, no one needs to expose themselves to excess levels of sunlight, beyond the amount needed to avoid vitamin D deficiency.

56. A. laid	**B.** lay	**C.** lied	**D.** lie
57. A. effected	**B.** contracted	**C.** affected	**D.** coughed
58. A. usually	**B.** naturally	**C.** ordinarily	**D.** normally
59. A. protect	**B.** prevent	**C.** prohibit	**D.** probe
60. A. variable	**B.** variables	**C.** variably	**D.** variability
61. A. undertake	**B.** undertaken	**C.** undergo	**D.** underwent
62. A. belong to	**B.** pertain to	**C.** belonging to	**D.** pertaining to
63. A. looking at	**B.** looking for	**C.** looking into	**D.** looking out
64. A. involved	**B.** involve	**C.** solved	**D.** solve
65. A. averted	**B.** avoided	**C.** shunned	**D.** eluded

III Writing

 ## Question 66

- Write about the following topic.

  Doctor is a respected profession, and the practitioners shoulder important social responsibility. What defines a qualified doctor?
- Write an essay of no less than 150 words on your answer sheet.

医护英语水平考试（三级）
模拟训练（五）
Medical English Test System（METS）Level 3

Ⅰ Listening

Part One >>>>>>

 Questions 1—5

- You will hear five extracts from conversations taking place in different clinical departments.
- Choose which case each doctor is discussing from the list **A—F**.
- Use each letter **A—F** only once. There is one extra letter which you **DO NOT** need to use.
- Mark the corresponding letter on your **answer sheet**.
- You will hear each extract twice.

| Doctor 1 | | 1 |

| Doctor 2 | | 2 |

| Doctor 3 | | 3 |

| Doctor 4 | | 4 |

| Doctor 5 | | 5 |

A. The patient took calcium supplements six months ago.

B. The patient is diagnosed with cholecystitis.

C. The patient's physiologic status meets the criteria of remote or no chance for recovery.

D. The patient has some problem with his bowel.

E. The patient is a smoker.

F. The patient is taking antibiotics.

Part Two >>>>>>

Questions 6—13

- You will hear a conversation between a reporter and a cardiologist.
- For each of the following statements, decide whether it is **True (A)** or **False (B)**. If there is not enough information to answer **True (A)** or **False (B)**, choose **Not Given (C)**.
- Mark the corresponding letter on your **answer sheet**.
- You will hear the recording twice.

6. In the USA, now physically active jobs make up less than 10% of workforce.
   A. True   B. False   C. Not Given

7. Sitting for long periods may cause heart disease.
   A. True   B. False   C. Not Given

8. Dr. Michos is physically active and leads a completely healthy lifestyle.
   A. True   B. False   C. Not Given

9. High levels of exercise can reduce the risk of heart disease.
   A. True   B. False   C. Not Given

10. People with high levels of activity have no cardiovascular risk.
    A. True   B. False   C. Not Given

11. Dr. Michos attends some meetings which are held outside rooms.
    A. True   B. False   C. Not Given

12. People who have to be sitting in front of the computer all day can break up the time.
    A. True   B. False   C. Not Given

13. According to Dr. Michos, 11,000 steps a day is recommended.
    A. True   B. False   C. Not Given

Part Three >>>>>>

Questions 14—20

- You will hear a discussion among an instructor and two medical students.
- For questions **14—20**, choose the most appropriate answer.
- Mark the corresponding letter on your **answer sheet**.

- You will hear the discussion twice.

---

14. Cellulitis is a bacterial infection of the _____.
  A. skin   **B.** cell   **C.** lung

15. A break in the skin can be caused by the following EXCEPT _____.
  A. burns   **B.** grazes   **C.** swelling

16. The symptoms for cellulitis include the following EXCEPT _____.
  A. inflammation of the affected area
  B. inflammation of lymph glands
  C. blisters, skin dimpling, or spots

17. To prevent cellulitis, we should do the following EXCETP _____.
  A. reducing the likelihood of scratching the skin
  B. avoid using of moisturizers
  C. avoid being overweight

18. Which of the following statements about cellulitis treatment is true?
  A. Cellulitis can be treated at home.
  B. Cellulitis requires no treatment.
  C. Cellulitis needs to be treated by a doctor.

19. Some people have suggested using tea tree oil for treatment because they may have _____.
  A. antibacterial   **B.** antibody   **A.** antidote

20. Which of the following statements about cellulitis is **NOT** true?
  A. There is no evidence that garlic can treat cellulitis.
  B. Coconut oil can be used to treat cellulitis.
  C. Without timely treatment, cellulitis can be life-threatening.

Part Four >>>>>>

Questions 21—25

- You will hear a speech on natural ways to adjust sleeping habits.
- Complete the notes. In each blank, write only one word.
- Write the answers on your **answer sheet**.
- You will hear the speech twice.

Notes:

There are easy, natural fixes that can improve your sleep.

- Warm (**21**) _____, chamomile tea and tart cherry juice are recommended for patients with sleep trouble.
- Moderate (**22**) _____ exercise boosts the amount of deep sleep you get.
  Endorphins released by exercises keep people awake and raise core body temperature.
- Melatonin supplements is a (**23**) _____ released in the brain for sleepiness.
  Exposure to unnatural light prevents melatonin release.
  Melatonin is available at local pharmacies as an over-the-counter supplement.
  You are recommended to consistently buy the same brand of melatonin supplements.
- Between 65 and 72 degrees is the ideal temperature.
  Women who are going through (**24**) _____ and hot flashes should keep the room cool.
- You are recommended to use a flashlight at night for less visual (**25**) _____.

II Reading

Part One >>>>>>

Questions 26—35

- Read the following passage about an outbreak of salmonella.

Egg Farm Responsible for Salmonella Outbreak

1 Perhaps more disturbing, the report says, is that "unacceptable rodent activity" had been going on at the facility for months before the first of the salmonella-related illnesses occurred, but the facility's management did not take appropriate actions and unsanitary practices continued. Thirty-five people who consumed eggs traced back to Rose Acre Farms' facility in Hyde County, North Carolina, have been sick since last November, the Centers for Disease Control and Prevention said. The inspection described in the report was conducted from late March to mid-April, in response to the outbreak of illness.

2 Last month, Rose Acre Farms, one of the biggest egg producers in the country, recalled nearly 207 million eggs because of fears they have been contaminated with salmonella. In a statement, the family-owned company apologized to those who "may have been sickened" and said it has taken "numerous remedial actions" and other steps "to ensure the farm meets or exceeds" federal standards. Rose Acre Farms takes food safety and the welfare of our hens, workers and consumers very seriously. "We responsibly follow the requirements of the FDA's(Food and Drug Administration) Egg Safety Rule, the Food Safety Modernization Act and the Food and Drug and Cosmetic Act because we care about providing safe, nutritious and affordable eggs," the Seymour, Indiana-based company said. "When we fall short of expectations, we're disappointed in ourselves and we strive to correct any problems and institute safeguards that ensure those problems won't occur again. We vow to do better in the future."

3 The report says that rodent infestation had been a problem at the company's Rose Acre Farms since at least last September. By late March and early April after several people had already been sick, an inspector visited the facility multiple times and found dozens of rodents running around rows of poultry houses. A few carcasses were found lying in and outside the houses. Sanitation procedures were also neither implemented nor followed, the report says. Employees were seen touching their faces, hair, buttocks and dirty surfaces, and then handling food without changing gloves or washing their hands. Production equipment were covered in dirt and food debris and were unclean for multiple days during the inspection. One employee was seen cleaning equipment with a steel wool scrubber that had been stored on a cart in a dustpan with a pool of dirty water. Condensation was also seen dripping from ceilings, pipes, and walls onto production equipment.

4 The "unsanitary conditions and poor employee practices" created an environment allowed for pathogens that could cause egg contamination to thrive throughout the facility, the report says. 200 million eggs recalled because of salmonella concerns. "The worst thing about it wasn't like this was news to Rose Acre Farms when the FDA got out there," said Jory Lange, a Houston-based attorney representing a woman who was infected with salmonella. "If Rose Acre Farms had just taken actions last year, there might not have been a salmonella outbreak." "The problem with rodents in a facility that's making food is that they spread pathogens and pathogens can be deadly," added Lange, who specializes in food-safety litigation. "So whatever it takes to get rid of them, you've got to get rid of them. Otherwise, you're endangering the public." The Hyde County facility produces 2.3 million eggs a day from 3 million hens. Eggs produced at the farm are distributed to retail stores and restaurants in Colorado, Florida, New Jersey, New York, Pennsylvania, Virginia, West Virginia and the Carolinas. Illnesses have been reported in all those states, the majority of which were from New York and Virginia, the CDC said.

5 Salmonella can come from contaminated animal products such as beef, poultry, milk and eggs, as well as fruits and vegetables. It can cause fever, diarrhea, nausea, vomiting and abdominal pain among healthy people, but can lead to fatal infections among children younger than 5, adults older than 65 and those with weak immune systems. Salmonella causes about 1.2 million illnesses, 23,000 hospitalizations and 450 deaths every year in the United States, according to the CDC. While most recover completely, some people suffer from long-term effects such as reactive arthritis, which is joint pain and swelling caused by infection.

 ## Questions 26—30

- Choose the most appropriate subheading from the list A—F for each paragraph.
- Use each letter **A—F** only once. There is one extra letter which you **DO NOT** need to use.
- Mark the corresponding letter on your answer sheet.

26. Paragraph 1 _____

27. Paragraph 2 _____

28. Paragraph 3 _____

29. Paragraph 4 _____

30. Paragraph 5 _____

A. Unsanitary and irregular practices found by an inspector at the egg farm existing rodent infestation.

B. Apologies and promises made by the Indiana—based company.

C. Outbreak of salmonella—related illnesses caused by rodent infection at an egg farm.

D. Source of Salmonella and damages it made to the body.

E. Unsanitary and irregular practices being the major causes of large—scaled egg contamination with pathogens.

F. Possible long—term effect made by salmonella.

 ## Questions 31—35

- Fill in each blank with the correct answer from the list **A—F**.
- Use each letter **A—F** only once. There is one extra letter which you **DO NOT** need to use.
- Mark the corresponding letter on your **answer sheet.**

31. Until the first salmonella related illness occurred, the management of the facility had not yet taken _____ and improved unhygienic practices.

32. We're _____ ourselves and we strive to correct any problems and institute safeguards that ensure those problems won't occur again.

33. A few carcasses were found _____ and outside the houses.

34. Eggs produced at the farm are _____ retail stores and restaurants in Colorado, Florida, New Jersey, New York, Pennsylvania, Virginia, West Virginia and the Carolinas.

35. Salmonella can come from _____ such as beef, poultry, milk and eggs, as well as fruits and vegetables.

> **A.** appropriate actions
> **B.** contaminated animal products
> **C.** disappointed in
> **D.** lying in
> **E.** coming from
> **F.** distributed to

Part Two >>>>>>

Questions 36—42

- Read the following passage about Alzheimer's disease.
- Choose the best answer **A, B, C** or **D.**
- Mark the corresponding letter on your **answer sheet.**

Alzheimer's Disease and Its Causes

Dame Barbara Windsor, one of the most recognizable faces in Britain known for her roles in Eastenders and the "Carry On" films, has been diagnosed with Alzheimer's disease, her husband has revealed.

She is one of around 850,000 people suffering with some form of dementia in the UK.

The majority have Alzheimer's disease, a terminal condition affecting the brain which the 80-year-old was diagnosed with four years ago.

The following are some fast facts about Alzheimer's disease.

What is Alzheimer's disease?

Alzheimer's disease is the most common cause of dementia, which is a collective term for symptoms including problems with language and thinking, and commonly memory loss. The hallmark of the disease is the build-up in the brain of damaging clumps of proteins, known as "plaques" and "tangles". These buildups gradually kill the junctions between nerve cells in the brain, known as synapses, and eventually strangle the neurons themselves leading to the death of brain tissue. Brains of people with Alzheimer's also have much lower levels of neurotransmitter chemicals like acetylcholine, which are another important part of brain signals.

What causes Alzheimer's?

This is still poorly understood. Scientists do not fully know what triggers the build-up of these plaques and whether they're a symptom or cause of the disease. However there are several factors which increase the risk, with age being the biggest, one sufferer in 20 is less risk than that under the age of 65 and early onset forms of the disease can strike from around 40.

Lifestyle factors including smoking, obesity and diet are another major factor in increasing risk, and suffering a head injury, including a minor concussion, can increase the risk by as much as two-thirds. There are twice as many women with Alzheimer's over the age 65 as men and the reason for this is also not fully understood. There are also some inherited genetic risks, and other health conditions such as having a learning disability can increase your chances of suffering from the disease.

What are its symptoms?

In many cases, the disease takes a long time to develop and can go unnoticed in older relatives making supportive treatment hard to deliver. Often the first recognized symptoms are once-routine tasks such as preparing a meal or taking a trip to shops become more difficult. People with the disease may get lost more easily or forget key dates or the names and faces of relatives. Depression can be a very early sign which may occur before any physical hallmarks in the brain. In later stages people can become non-verbal and it can cause large swings in behavior leading to aggression and other behaviors which make caring for them at home more difficult.

Is there a cure?

There is no cure for the disease, though it is a major research area along with developing tests for earlier diagnosis. Support is usually focused on coming to terms with the diagnosis and adapting lifestyle and care arrangements to maximize quality of life, as well as teaching coping strategies for memory. There are drug treatments which can temporarily improve some symptoms. In earlier stages drugs like Exelon or Reminy can improve memory problems and concentration, typically by addressing the imbalances in neurotransmitter chemicals like acetylcholine. In later stages drug treatments can help to address some of the more challenging symptoms such as delusions or aggression.

36. What is Alzheimer's disease?

    A. Alzheimer's disease is the most common cause of dementia, which is a collective term for symptoms including problems with language and thinking, and commonly memory loss.

    B. Alzheimer's disease is the most common cause of dementia, which is a collective term for symptoms including problems with language and commonly memory loss.

    C. Alzheimer's disease is the most common cause of dementia, which is a collective term for symptoms including problems with thinking and commonly memory loss.

    D. Alzheimer's disease is the most common cause of dementia, which is a collective term for symptoms including problems with commonly memory loss.

37. What causes Alzheimer's?

    A. Build-up of plaques.

    B. The aging process.

    C. The cause is poorly understood.

    D. Early onset of strokes.

38. What kind of people are more susceptible to Alzheimer's disease?

    A. The young people are more likely to develop Alzheimer's disease.

    B. Males are more likely to develop Alzheimer's disease.

    C. Adults are more likely to develop Alzheimer's disease.

    D. The aged are more likely to develop Alzheimer's disease.

39. What lifestyle factors can lead to increased risk of Alzheimer?

    A. Lifestyle factors including sleeping and diet are major factors in increasing risk.

    B. Lifestyle factors including smoking, obesity and diet are major factors in increasing risk.

    C. Lifestyle factors including obesity and diet are major factors in increasing risk.

    D. Lifestyle factors including fruit and diet are major factors in increasing risk.

40. Which of the following statements about the symptoms of Alzheimer's is NOT true?

    A. The first symptom to be found is that the once-routine tasks, become more difficult.

    B. Depression can be a very late sign that comes after any physical feature of the brain.

    C. In later stages the affected individuals may have problems in oral communication.

    D. People with Alzheimer's may become aggressive.

41. Which of the following statements about the cure for Alzheimer's is true?

    A. It is a major research area along with developing tests for screening.

    B. It is a major research area along with developing tests for prognosis.

    C. It is a major research area along with developing tests for earlier prevention.

    D. It is a major research area along with developing tests for diagnosis.

42. According to the passage, which of the following statements is true about the treatment of Alzheimer's disease?

    A. The radical treatment is teaching coping strategies for memory.

B. There are drug treatments which can temporarily improve some symptoms.

C. Drugs like Exelon or Reminy can improve memory problems and concentration.

D. Drugs like Exelon or Reminy can address symptoms such as aggression.

Part Three >>>>>>

 ### Questions 43—50

- Read the following passage about American ginseng berry and colorectal cancer.
- For each of the following statements, decide whether it is **True (A)** or **False (B)**. If there is not enough information to answer **True (A)** or **False (B)**, choose **Not Given (C)**.
- Mark the corresponding letter on your **answer sheet**.

American Ginseng Berry Enhances Chemo Preventive Effect of 5-FU on Human Colorectal Cancer Cells

Colorectal cancer is one of the most common malignancies and ranks as the second greatest cause of cancer death in both men and women worldwide. Although early stage colorectal cancer can be cured by surgical resection, surgery is often combined with adjuvant radiotherapy and chemo-therapy with one or more chemotherapeutic agents. Even with effective strategies that continue to be developed for treating colorectal cancer, chemotherapy has the drawbacks of severe adverse effects and dose-limiting toxicity. Drug-related adverse events not only worsen patients' quality of life, but can also lead to their refusal to continue chemotherapy.

Chemotherapy-induced toxicity can be reduced by chemo-adjuvant compounds that potentiate tumoricidal effects with lower doses. Identifying non-toxic chemo-adjuvants among herbal medicines may be an essential step in advancing the treatment of cancer. Due to the increase in the consumption of herbal remedies in the United States along with a staggering popularity of the ginseng herb as a method of sustaining good health, significant focus has been placed on American ginseng (Panaxquinquefolius L.), which belongs to the genus Panax L. in the Araliaceae family. American ginseng has been reported to have stress-relieving qualities, anti-aging effects and digestion-aiding effects. Cancer treatment with botanicals like American ginseng has also received increasing attention in recent years. The major active components of ginseng are ginsenosides, a diverse group of steroid saponins. Ginsenosides are distributed in many parts of the ginseng plant, including the root, leaf and berry. The most commonly used part of the plant is the root, which is harvested in late summer to fall between its fourth and seventh years.

It is well documented that American ginseng berry extract (AGBE) could improve diabetic conditions, such as decreasing the blood glucose and body weight in mice, attenuating oxidant stress in cardiomyocytes, reducing chemotherapy-induced nausea/vomiting, and exerting antiproliferative activity against human breast carcinoma cells. Previously, our laboratory analyzed ginsenoside compounds in AGBE with different processing methods, and pilot data showed the effects on colorectal carcinoma cells. However, the mechanism of the antiproliferative effect of AGBE is not known. The 5-Fluorouracil (5-FU) is one of the most widely used chemotherapeutic agents in first-line therapy for colorectal cancer, and an overall survival benefit after fluorouracil-based chemotherapy has been firmly established. But for the treatment of metastatic colon cancer, however, higher 5-FU doses produced more adverse effects while not necessarily being more effective than lower doses. Therefore, if decreasing the dose of chemotherapy and increasing its anti-cancer effect could be accomplished by combining 5-FU with other agents, patients may benefit. However, chemotherapy with 5-FU and herbal medicines has rarely been studied.

Thus, this study investigated the potential synergistic tumoricidal effects of AGBE on 5-FU. We used various human colorectal cancer cell lines, SW-480, HCT-116 and HT-29, which have undergone extensive laboratory cancer research and have been the models for the cellular pathways studies of chemotherapy on cancer cells. Furthermore, we observed the combined effect on cell apoptosis, cell cycle and cycle A in SW-480 cells to elucidate the possible mechanism in these cells. This is an important preliminary step in the development of an effective chemo. The successful treatment regimens for cancer include combination chemotherapy, which is often more effective than single chemotherapy because of additive or synergistic effects.

In the present study, we evaluated the effects of AGBE in enhancing the chemopreventive efficacy of 5-FU on human colorectal cancer cells. Our data suggest that AGBE has the potential to heighten the tumoricidal effects of 5-FU and that 5-FU-induced antiproliferation of human colorectal cancer cells can be strengthened by combination with AGBE. The mechanism may include the enhancement of AGBE on the Sand G2/M phases arrest and the expression level of cyclin A, but not the induction of cell apoptosis.

43. Colorectal cancer is considered as the top cause of cancer death in both men and women worldwide.

    A. True   **B.** False   **C.** Not Given

44. It has been reported that American ginseng can be used to relieve stress retard the aging process, and aid digetion.

    A. True   **B.** False   **C.** Not Given

45. The 5-Fluorouracil (5-FU) is one of the most widely used chemotherapeutic agents in first-line therapy for colorectal cancer.

    A. True   **B.** False   **C.** Not Given

46. The concentrations of ginsenoside compounds vary significantly depending on genetics, season, geographical distribution, plant growth, and production and extract processes.

A. True   **B.** False   **C.** Not Given

47. It is not clear whether consuming AGBE with chemotherapy affects the efficacy of chemotherapeutic agents.

A. True   **B.** False   **C.** Not Given

48. Because of additive or synergistic effects combination chemotherapy is often less effetine than single chemotherapy.

A. True   **B.** False   **C.** Not Given

49. The 5-FU induced antiproliferation of human colorectal cancer cells may be weakened by combination with AGBE.

A. True   **B.** False   **C.** Not Given

50. The mechanism of AGBE's potential to heighten the turmoricidal effects of 5-FU has nothing to do with the induction of cell apoptosis.

A. True   **B.** False   **C.** Not Given

Part Four >>>>>>

 ## Questions 51—55

- Read the following passage about physical health. Five sentences have been removed from the passage.
- Fill in each blank with the most appropriate sentence from the list **A—F**. There is one extra sentence which you **DO NOT** need to use.
- Mark the corresponding letter on your **answer sheet.**

Optimism and Physical Health

Few outcomes are more important than staying alive, and optimism is linked to life longevity. Maruta, Colligan, Malinchoc, and Offord (2000) examined whether explanatory styles served as risk factors for early death. With a large longitudinal sample collected in the mid-1960s, the researchers categorized medical patients as optimistic, mixed, or pessimistic. Optimism was operationalized using parts of the Minnesota Multiphasic Personality Inventory. (**51**) _____

Considering that, for a middle-aged person of average health, the difference between sudden death risk factors for smokers and non-smokers is 5%—10%, the protective effect of optimism found in this study is massive.

Optimism also plays a role in the recovery from illness and disease. (**52**) _____

These studies have found that optimistic people experience less distress when faced with potentially life-threatening cancer diagnoses. For example, Schou and colleagues (2005) found that a superior "fighting spirit" found in optimists predicted substantially better quality of life one year after breast cancer surgery. In this case, optimism appeared to protect against an urge to withdraw from social activities, which may be important for healing. People who tend to be more optimistic and more mindful had an increase in sleep quality. (**53**) _____ A sample of middle-aged women was tested for precursors to atherosclerosis at a baseline three years later.

Optimism can have an effect on a person's immune system, as well. In one study, elderly adults were immunized for influenza. Two weeks later, their immune response to the vaccination was measured. Greater optimism predicted greater antibody production and better immune outcomes. Five studies have also investigated optimism and disease progression in people infected with HIV. This study examined a sample of entering law students over five time points in their first year of law school. Dispositional optimism (the tendency to be generally optimistic about your life) and optimism about law school, in particular, were assessed, along with measures of positive and negative affect (to determine whether any relationships between optimism and immune system functioning could be better explained through positive or negative affect). This study found that optimism predicted superior cell-mediated immunity, an important part of the immune system's response to infectious agents. Furthermore, negative affect did not predict changes in immune function. (**54**) _____

Thus, it appears that an optimistic outlook appears not only to be strongly positively related to a healthy immune system but also to better outcomes for people with compromised immune systems.

Optimism has also been investigated in health-related behaviors. In examining the risk of developing alcohol dependence, one study found that optimism protected against drinking problems in people with a family history of alcoholism. As family history is one of the greatest risk factors for developing substance dependence, optimism's protective effects against its influence may be very important for public health efforts. Beyond helping to prevent substance use problems from developing, optimism may predict better outcomes from efforts to quit using. Pregnant women who are higher in optimism have been shown to be less likely to abuse substances while pregnant.

(**55**) _____ The mere act of expecting positive outcomes and being hopeful can boost a person's immune system, protect against harmful behaviors, prevent chronic disease, and help people cope following troubling news. Optimism can even predict a longer life. Among psychological constructs, optimism may be one of the most important predictors of physical health.

A. Multiple studies have investigated the role of optimism in people undergoing treatment for cancer.

B. The studies described above share a common theme: optimism can have profound effects on a person's physical health.

C. What this means is that optimism appears to have a unique value among the factors that compose a person's immune system.

D. The researchers found that for every 10 points increase in a person's score on their optimism scale, the risk of early death decreased by 19%.

E. There is also evidence that optimism can protect against the development of chronic diseases.

F. Optimists are also able to recover from disappointments more quickly by attending to positive outcomes to a greater extent than negative ones.

Part Five >>>>>>

 Questions 56—65

- Read the following passage about kidney transplantation.
- Fill in each blank with the correct choice **A, B, C** or **D.**
- Mark the corresponding letter on your **answer sheet.**

Kidney Transplantation

Kidney transplantation or renal transplantation is the organ transplant of a kidney into a patient with end-stage renal disease. Kidney transplantation is (**56**) _____ classified as deceased-donor or living-donor transplantation depending on the source of the donor organ.

One of the earliest mentions about the real possibility of a kidney transplant was by American medical researcher Simon Flexner, who declared in a reading of his paper on "Tendencies in Pathology" in the University of Chicago in 1907 that it would be possible in the then-future for diseased human organs substitution for healthy ones by surgery, including arteries, stomach, kidneys and heart. Occasionally, the kidney is (**57**) _____ together with the pancreas. University of Minnesota surgeons Richard and William Kelly perform the first successful simultaneous pancreas-kidney transplant in the world in 1966. This is done in patients with diabetes mellitus type 1, in whom the diabetes is due to destruction of the beta cells of the pancreas and in whom the diabetes has caused renal failure. This is almost always a deceased donor transplant. Only (**58**) _____ living donor pancreas transplants have been done. For individuals with diabetes and renal failure, the advantages of earlier transplant from a living donor are far superior to the risks of continued dialysis until a combined kidney and pancreas are available from a deceased donor. A patient can either receive a living kidney followed by a donor pancreas at a later date or a combined kidney-pancreas from a donor.

Transplanting just the islet cells from the pancreas is still in the experimental stage, but shows promise. This involves taking a deceased donor pancreas, breaking it down, and extracting the islet cells that make insulin. The cells are then injected through a catheter into the recipient and they generally lodge in the liver. The recipient still needs to take immune suppressants to avoid rejection, but no surgery is required. Most people need two or three such injections, and many are not completely insulin-free. Kidney transplantation is a life-extending procedure. The typical patient will live 10 to 15 years longer with a kidney transplant than being kept on dialysis. The increase in longevity is greater for (**59**) _____ patients, but even 75-year-old recipients gain an average of four more years of life. People generally have more energy, a less restricted diet, and fewer complications with a kidney transplant than if they stay on conventional dialysis.

Some studies seem to suggest that the longer a patient is on dialysis before the transplant, the less time the kidney will last. It is not clear why this occurs, but it underscores the need for rapid referral to a transplant program. Ideally, a kidney transplant should be pre-emptive, i. e. , take place before the patient begins dialysis. The reason why kidneys fail over time after transplantation has been elucidated in recent years. (**60**) _____ recurrence of the original kidney disease, also rejection and progressive scarring play a decisive role. Avoiding rejection by strict medication adherence is of utmost importance to avoid failure of the kidney transplant.

In addition to nationality, transplantation rates differ based on race, sex, and income. A study done with patients beginning long-term dialysis showed that the socio-demographic barriers to renal transplantation are relevant even before patients are on the transplant list. For example, different socio-demographic groups express different interest and complete pre-transplant (**61**) _____ at different rates. Previous (**62**) _____ to create fair transplantation policies have focused on patients currently on the transplantation waiting list.

The attainment of tolerance (**63**) _____ a highly desirable goal in recipients of kidney transplants. Achievement of this goal would extend graft survival and eradicate toxicities related to long-term immunosuppression. Mechanistic studies of spontaneously tolerant kidney transplant recipients have (**64**) _____ potential roles for B or regulatory T cells, or both, in the maintenance of tolerance. Mixed hematopoietic chimerism has been the most commonly used approach to induce tolerance. Distinct protocols at three major transplant centers have (**65**) _____ successful withdrawal of immunosuppression in a subset of living donor kidney transplant recipients at the expense of complications such as infections and graft versus host disease. The addition of regulatory cell therapies to tolerance induction protocols could enhance success while minimizing complications. This review summarizes the features of spontaneous tolerance in kidney transplant recipients, the results of clinical trials of tolerance induction in the context of living donor kidney transplant, and potential measures to improve the safety and efficacy of tolerance induction strategies.

56. A. typical   **B.** atypical   **C.** typically   **D.** atypically

57. A. transplant   **B.** transplanted   **C.** remove   **D.** removed

58. A. a few   **B.** few   **C.** little   **D.** a little

59. A. old   **B.** older   **C.** young   **D.** younger

60. A. Away from   **B.** Far from   **C.** Apart from   **D.** Suffer from

61. A. workup   **B.** work out   **C.** workout   **D.** work up

62. A. successes   **B.** efforts   **C.** achievements   **D.** struggles

63. A. remain   **B.** remains   **C.** keep   **D.** kept

64. A. covered   **B.** cover   **C.** covering   **D.** uncovered

65. A. led to   **B.** resulted to   **C.** brought to   **D.** gave to

III Writing

 ## Question 66

- Write about the following topic.

  In recent years, the doctor-patient relationship has become increasingly tense and complicated, and the disputes between doctors and patients are becoming worse. Medical activities and the normal order of hospitals are deeply affected. Please give some suggestions of improving the doctor-patient relationship.

- Write an essay of no less than 150 words on your answer sheet.

医护英语水平考试（三级）

模拟训练（六）

Medical English Test System（METS）
Level 3

Ⅰ Listening

Part One >>>>>>

Questions 1—5

- You will hear five extracts from conversations taking place in different clinical departments.
- Choose which case each doctor is discussing from the list **A—F**.
- Use each letter **A—F** only once. There is one extra letter which you **DO NOT** need to use.
- Mark the corresponding letter on your **answer sheet**.
- You will hear each extract twice.

Doctor 1 ⬜ 1

Doctor 2 ⬜ 2

Doctor 3 ⬜ 3

Doctor 4 ⬜ 4

Doctor 5 ⬜ 5

A. The patient has an early lung tumor.

B. The patient is not recommended to take hormone therapy.

C. The patient is advised to have the surgery immediately.

D. The patient is pregnant.

E. The patient has some problem with his pancreas.

F. The patient has kidney disease.

Part Two >>>>>>

Questions 6—13

- You will hear a conversation between a reporter and a transplantation expert.
- For each of the following statements, decide whether it is **True (A)** or **False (B)**. If there is not enough information to answer **True (A)** or **False (B)**, choose **Not Given (C)**.
- Mark the corresponding letter on your **answer sheet**.
- You will hear the recording twice.

---

6. More than 20 people die each day from lack of a transplant.
   A. True   **B.** False   **C.** Not Given

7. Living donors must have a body mass index that is more than 35.
   A. True   **B.** False   **C.** Not Given

8. Living donors can donate one of their kidneys and part of their liver.
   A. True   **B.** False   **C.** Not Given

9. For kidney donors, drinking a large amount of water after the surgery is good for recovery.
   A. True   **B.** False   **C.** Not Given

10. Living donation has no influence on life expectancy.
    A. True   **B.** False   **C.** Not Given

11. People having a medical condition cannot donate their organs.
    A. True   **B.** False   **C.** Not Given

12. Organ donors can receive a sum of money for postoperative care.
    A. True   **B.** False   **C.** Not Given

13. Buying or selling organs is illegal in the USA.
    A. True   **B.** False   **C.** Not Given

Part Three >>>>>>

Questions 14—20

- You will hear a discussion among an instructor and two medical students.
- For questions **14—20**, choose the best appropriate answer.
- Mark the corresponding letter on your **answer sheet**.

- You will hear the discussion twice.

---

14. How many new cases of breast cancer were diagnosed in 2012?

    A. 1. 6 million   **B.** 1. 7 million   **C.** 1. 8 million

15. Breast cancer risk _____ each decade until menopause.

    A. increases   **B.** levels off   **C.** decreases

16. Generally, survival rates for breast cancer worldwide _____.

    A. have increased   **B.** have leveled off   **C.** have decreased

17. The survival rate for breast cancer diagnosed at advanced stage is _____.

    A. 80 percent   **B.** 90 percent   **C.** 24 percent

18. Risk factors for breast cancer include the following EXCEPT _____.

    A. early menarche

    B. late natural menopause

    C. first pregnancy over the age of 40

19. Hormone therapy containing _____ increases risk.

    A. androgen   **B.** oestrogen   **C.** testosterone

20. Which country had the second highest rate of breast cancer in 2012?

    A. Belgium   **B.** Denmark   **C.** Netherlands

Part Four >>>>>

Questions 21—25

- You will hear a speech on strategies for dementia.
- Complete the notes. In each blank, write only one word.
- Write the answers on your **answer sheet**.
- You will hear the speech twice.

Notes:

There are some strategies that you need to consider after you or your families receive a dementia diagnosis:

- Allow yourself time to adjust, be gentle and (**21**) _____ with yourself, and try to feel all the feelings.
- Set up routines and expectations.
- Find an experienced dementia care (**22**) _____ because when caregivers and people with dementia sought treatment for depression, they gained greater access to care, services and support.

- Give each other space.

  Most people with dementia develop behavioral symptoms or (**23**) _____ problems at some point during their illness.

- Pace yourself.

  Keep the day structured and (**24**) _____ , the environment uncluttered and activities simple.

- Make time for daily exercise.

  A daily walk can be an effective (**25**) _____ and antianxiety remedy.

Ⅱ Reading

Part One >>>>>>

 Questions 26—35

- Read the following passage about mobile phone and health.

Mobile Phone and Health

1 Can talking on a mobile phone be hazardous to your health? It is difficult to know for sure. Some research suggests that heavy users of mobile phones are at a greater risk of developing cancerous brain tumors. However, many other studies suggest there are no links between cancer and mobile phone use.

2 The main problem with the current research is that mobile phones have only been popular since the 1990s. As a result, it is impossible to study long-term exposure to mobile phones. This concerns many health professionals who point out that certain cancers can take over twenty years to develop. Another concern about these studies is that many have been funded by the mobile phone industry or benefit from it.

3 Over five billion people now use mobile phones on a daily basis, and many talk for more than an hour a day. Mobile phone antennas are similar to microwave ovens. While both rely on electromagnetic radiation (EMR), the radio waves in mobile phones are lower in frequency. Microwave ovens have radio wave frequencies that are high enough to cook food, and they are also known to be dangerous to human tissues like those in the brain. The concern is that the lower-frequency radio waves that mobile phones rely on may also be dangerous. It seems logical that holding a heat source near your brain for a long period of time is a potential health hazard.

4 Some researchers believe that other types of wireless technology may also be dangerous to human health, including cordless phones, wireless gaming consoles, and laptop or tablet computers with wireless connections. They suggest replacing all cordless and wireless devices with wired ones where possible. They also say that many cordless phones can emit dangerous levels of electromagnetic radiation even when they are not in use. They even suggest keeping electronic devices such as desk-top and tablet computers out of the bedroom, or at least six feet from the head while we're sleeping.

5 A growing number of health professionals worldwide are recommending that mobile phone users err on the side of caution until more definitive studies can be conducted. They use the example of tobacco to illustrate the potential risks. Many years ago, people smoked freely and were not concerned about the effects of cigarettes on their health. Today, people know that cigarettes cause lung cancer, though it is still unknown exactly how or why. Some doctors fear that the same thing will happen with mobile phones. In May 2016, the UK's *Independent* newspaper reported on research by the US government's National Toxicology Program that showed a slight increase in brain tumours among rats exposed to the type of radio frequencies commonly emitted by mobile phones. This doesn't prove that mobile phones can cause brain tumours in humans, but it does show that it's possible. As a result, many experts now recommend texting or using head sets or speaker phones instead of holding a mobile phone to the ear.

 Questions 26—30

- Choose the most appropriate subheading from the list **A—F** for each paragraph.
- Use each letter **A—F** only once. There is one extra letter which you **DO NOT** need to use.
- Mark the corresponding letter on your **answer sheet**.

26. Paragraph 1 _____

27. Paragraph 2 _____

28. Paragraph 3 _____

29. Paragraph 4 _____

30. Paragraph 5 _____

A. Advice from researchers about the use of electronic devices.

B. Potential health hazard brought by radio wave frequencies.

C. Two conflicting research results about whether there is a link between using mobile phone and cancer.

D. Close relationship between mobile phone and people's health.

E. More evidence to prove the possible development of brain tumor caused by radio frequencies from mobile phones.

F. Two concerns about the factors affecting the research results.

Questions 31—35

- Fill in each blank with the correct answer from the list **A—F**.
- Use each letter **A—F** only once. There is one extra letter which you **DO NOT** need to use.
- Mark the corresponding letter on your **answer sheet**.

31. According to some research, people who use mobile phones a lot have a _____ of developing cancerous brain tumours.

32. Research funded by mobile phone industry or researchers who _____ the research activity may be the factors affecting research results.

33. The worry is that the _____ radio waves that mobile phones depend on may also be hazardous.

34. Some researchers also point out that many cordless phones cansend out dangerous levels of _____ even when they are not used.

35. Therefore, many specialists now advise texting or using _____ or speaker phones instead of holding a mobile phone to the ear.

> **A.** lower-frequency
> **B.** electromagnetic radiation
> **C.** greater risk
> **D.** benefit from
> **E.** brain tumours
> **F.** head sets

Part Two >>>>>>

Questions 36—42

- Read the following passage from a news website.
- Choose the best answer **A, B, C** or **D**.
- Mark the corresponding letter on your **answer sheet**.

A grieving husband has described his shock at realizing his wife may have been among those whose lives were cut short due to a breast cancer screening error.

Health secretary Jeremy Hunt said a "computer algorithm failure" dating back to 2009 had meant many women aged between 68 and 71 in England were not invited to their final routine screening.

He said it was not currently known whether any delay in diagnosis resulted in avoidable death, but that it is estimated between 135 and 270 women had their lives shortened as a result.

Brian Gough said his wife never received a letter inviting her to go for routine screening in 2009—and that after she later found a lump, a scan in October 2010 revealed she had stage three breast cancer.

He said he was watching the television on Wednesday when the news of the screening error broke, leaving him "shell shocked".

He said he was convinced his wife was a victim of the "massive error" because her illness struck "right absolutely plum in the centre of when this happened".

Despite his shock, Mr. Gough said he admired the health secretary for "getting up and not trying to hide the truth".

"I am glad the truth has come out, and I just hope that people take more notice of these glitches," he said.

"Potentially we are talking about 450,000 women who could have died, it is all very well saying only a percentage but we are not born as a percentage of anything, we are a person."

Mr. Hunt faced questions about the speed with when women who have been affected by the mistake will be contacted, and was asked by Labour's Liz McInnes whether the alarm had been raised by GPs wondering why their patients had not been invited to a screening.

Mr. Hunt said: "I'm not aware of any such instances but that's exactly what we want to look at in this review.

"It does seem strange that people didn't come forward who were expecting to be invited and didn't get an invitation and that didn't set hares running, so that's one of the things we need to look at."

The health secretary apologized "wholeheartedly and unreservedly for the suffering caused" on behalf of the government, Public Health England and the NHS.

He told MPs that all those living in the UK who are registered with a GP would be contacted before the end of May, with the first 65,000 letters going out this week.

The letters will tell women under 72 they will automatically be sent an invitation to a catch-up screening, and those aged 72 and over will be given access to a helpline to decide whether a screening is appropriate for them.

Mr. Gough said that following her diagnosis, his wife Trixie underwent an operation, chemotherapy, radiotherapy and then scans every three months during which her cancer was under control.

But he said it returned again, prompting another two years of chemotherapy and treatment during what he described as an "horrendous situation".

He said his wife died three days after Christmas in 2015, and the 76-year-old never once complained during her cancer ordeal.

"She missed all of that because she didn't get diagnosed and she didn't know anything about it until a year ago," he said.

Mr. Gough believes that "maybe, just maybe" his wife might have come through the first lot of cancer treatment and survived if it had been diagnosed earlier.

36. What can be calculated as a result of breast cancer screening error?

    A. A grieving husband was shocked when he knew the truth.

    B. His wife died for the "computer algorithm failure".

    C. A lot of women had shortened their lives.

    D. Many women could avoid death without delay in diagnosis.

37. What made Brian Gough "shell shocked"?

    A. His wife didn't receive a letter for routine screening.

    B. His wife had stage three breast cancer.

    C. Something was wrong with screening.

    D. His wife could live longer without screening error.

38. Which of the following statements is NOT true?

    A. Mr. Gough's wife was a victim of breast cancer screening error.

    B. Jeremy Hunt told the fact about screening error.

    C. Thousands of women could have died due to screening error.

    D. All the women would be invited to a screening in order to correct the error.

39. Mr. Hunt wants to look at _____.

    A. why such mistakes didn't happen before

    B. why people didn't get invited to have a check up

    C. why people didn't move forward

    D. why people set hares running

40. According to the passage, Mr. Gough's wife _____.

    A. used chemical substances to treat her disease

    B. received the treatment of disease by exposure to a radioactive substance

    C. experienced a painful process of treatment

    D. all the above answers are correct

41. Mr. Gough was sad for his wife's death because of the following reasons EXCEPT that _____.

    A. his wife might have survived if her cancer had been diagnosed earlier

B. it was too late when his wife got diagnosed

C. he could be sure that his wife would recover with timely treatment

D. screening error was accountable for his wife's death

42. A proper title for this text could be _____.

    A. a grieving husband's memory of his wife

    B. a man's "shell shocked" about breast cancer screening error

    C. a woman patient's treatment experiences

    D. diagnosis and treatment of the breast cancer

Part Three >>>>>>

 ## Questions 43—50

- Read the following passage about anorexia nervous.
- For each of the following statements, decide whether it is **True (A)** or **False (B)**. If there is not enough information to answer **True (A)** or **False (B)**, choose **Not Given (C)**.
- Mark the corresponding letter on your **answer sheet**.

Anorexia Nervosa

Most people know about anorexia nervosa—when people deliberately starve themselves to keep their weight down—but bulimia, or excessive vomiting, is another extreme of the disorder.

Many people with anorexia see themselves as overweight even though they are in fact underweight. If asked they usually deny they have a problem with low weight. Often they weigh themselves frequently, eat only small amounts, and only eat certain foods.

Although bulimics have near normal weight, it comes at a price, and that is their health.

They delude themselves into thinking that the only way to keep the calories they have eaten from turning into fat is to make themselves vomit or by taking excessive amounts of laxatives.

What they don't realise is that it is not an effective way of preventing the absorption of extra calories.

It isn't just women who can suffer from anorexia or bulimia, although women are 10 times more liable to succumb to eating disorders.

Bulimia may start after months or years of anorexia. It is essentially a teenage problem, though it may extend into adult life or even begin then.

The frequent food binges by bulimics can lead to depression. The physical and psychiatric complications of his behaviour lead to educational, occupational, social and family problems.

One of the obvious signs of bulimia is hard skin or marks on the back of the hand due to repeated abrasion of the skin as the hand is thrust down the throat to produce vomiting.

A dentist may also spot the condition as the salivary glands can become enlarged as well as the teeth losing their enamel through repeated vomiting—which causes the teeth to come into contact with abnormal amounts of gastric acid.

And it is not just the outside appearance of the body that suffers.

Repeated vomiting also upsets the chemical balance of the blood, which can result in painful cramps, fits and even kidney damage.

A sympathetic ear is the first priority when it comes to treating the disorder.

Once the problem is out in the open, the sufferers and their doctors, friends and family can join together to fight it.

The person who have the disorder will need psychotherapy to tackle and overcome their behaviour. This will reveal why they feel they have to binge and vomit, and break the cycle.

There is help out there for anorexics and bulimics, but they must take the first step and seek help from their doctors as soon as possible before they seriously damage their health.

43. To lose weight, people with anorexia nervosa starve themselves on purpose.

    A. True   **B.** False   **C.** Not Given

44. Bulimics think that they can prevent themselves from absorbing extra calories by making themselves sick or taking laxatives beyond normal limits.

    A. True   **B.** False   **C.** Not Given

45. Female tend to succumb to eating disorders than male.

    A. True   **B.** False   **C.** Not Given

46. Eating too much food frequently is the direct reason for depression.

    A. True   **B.** False   **C.** Not Given

47. Because of abrasion of the skin many times, hard skin or marks will appear on the back of the hand as one of the signs of bulimia.

    A. True   **B.** False   **C.** Not Given

48. A sympathetic ear can treat the disorder.

A. True   **B.** False   **C.** Not Given

49. Nutritionists are very helpful for anorexics and bulimics, for they can give advice on what you should eat to remain healthy.

    A. True   **B.** False   **C.** Not Given

50. Seeing doctors as soon as possible is the first choice for anorexics and bulimics.

    A. True   **B.** False   **C.** Not Given

Part Four >>>>>>

 ## Questions 51—55

- Read the following passage about trans fat. Five sentences have been removed from the passage.
- Fill in each blank with the most appropriate sentence from the list **A—F**. There is one extra sentence which you **DO NOT** need to use.
- Mark the corresponding letter on your **answer sheet**.

Trans Fat

Does your mouth water when you think of cookies, donuts, burgers and French fries? Many people prefer junk food like these to healthy food because they develop a taste for it. Processed, baked, and fried foods often contain a high amount of trans fats.

Trans fat, or trans-unsaturated fatty acids, trans fatty acids, are a type of unsaturated fat that occur in small amounts in nature, but became widely produced industrially from vegetable fats for use in margarine, snack food, packaged baked goods, and frying fast food starting in the 1950s.

Trans fats raise bad cholesterol and lower the good cholesterol that your body needs. Fatty foods do more than cause obesity. (**51**) _____ People whose diet contains a high percentage of trans fats are at risk of developing heart disease or having a stroke.

Trans fat is a semi-solid type of oil. It is made by adding hydrogen to liquid oil. Food companies and restaurants choose to use trans fat oils because they're cheap and they make food like crackers and baked goods last longer. (**52**) _____ Trans fats became very popular in the second half of the 20th century. This is around the time butter got a bad name for its cholesterol levels. People were told to use margarine containing trans fats instead because it was "healthier", but we now know that butter is actually the healthier option.

Today doctors know how dangerous processed foods like margarine can be. In countries such as the US and Canada there are new government restrictions on food production. Food and beverage makers must attach a Nutrition Fact label to their products. **(53)** _____ In 2007 New York City banned trans fats from all restaurants, and according to recent studies this has prevented hundreds of heart attacks and strokes. Even fast food chains such as McDonalds are being forced to change their recipes as people become more health-conscious.

We all need some fat in our diet. There are three different types of fats: saturated fats, unsaturated fats and trans fats. Doctors recommend that we get most of our fatty calories from unsaturated fats. Neither butter nor margarine fits this category, though other spreads like peanut butter do. **(54)** _____ Another way is to avoid eating out, especially in fast food restaurants. Also, when shopping try to buy the majority of your food in the fresh-food section and limit the amount of processed and packaged food you buy. You might not think this is important if you're young, but the choices you make now will affect you for the rest of your life. **(55)** _____

In many countries, there are legal limits to trans fat content. Trans fats levels can be reduced or eliminated by using saturated fats such as lard, palm oil or fully hydrogenated fats, or by using interesterified fat. Other alternative formulations can also allow unsaturated fats to be used to replace saturated or partially hydrogenated fats.

A. Food manufacturers have voluntarily started using labels that clearly show how healthy each product is according to a simple rating system.

B. These labels list daily recommendations and details of all the ingredients in a product, including trans fats if they're used.

C. The healthier your diet is now, the longer and healthier your life will be.

D. Trans fats build up in the body and block blood flow to the heart.

E. Reading the list of ingredients on the label is a good way of avoiding dangerous ingredients like trans fats.

F. They also improve the taste and texture of food.

Part Five >>>>>>

 Questions 56—65

- Read the following passage about night cramp.
- Fill in each blank with the correct choice **A**, **B**, **C** or **D**.
- Mark the corresponding letter on your **answer sheet**.

Night Cramp

Night cramp is something from which a great many people occasionally suffer—and they don't easily forget it. Even the healthiest people may get a short, sharp pain in the legs after a(n) (**56**) _____ day.

Many older people can bring it on by making powerful stretching movements while lying down in bed. If this sort of night cramp becomes a real nuisance, (**57**) _____ over-stretching and taking tablets containing quinine sulphate at bed-time may be all that is needed.

A very small number of patients, however, cannot take quinine without becoming (**58**) _____ or getting buzzing in the ears. They may have to decide whether they would rather have cramp and no dizziness, or the reverse.

But cramp in the lower limbs in the daytime and in younger, active patients can be very distressing and is more (**59**) _____. It is not uncommon and has the rather clumsy name of intermittent claudications.

The patient first complains of aching legs after exercise. It may be slight, but gradually becomes more (**60**) _____. Then the pain is not merely an ache, but a definite, crippling cramp, which can become so severe that the patient finds he or she cannot (**61**) _____ after much walking.

Intermittent claudication is caused by the narrowing of the arteries and often starts in the 30s. It generally means that the arteries everywhere in the body have become narrowed and blood cannot reach the muscles fast enough when it is in use. The heart muscles may be equally (**62**) _____.

This condition may be a good enough excuse for not doing jobs you don't like but that is poor consolation. It is a disease which affects men far more than women and attacks are more common in cold weather, or even after sitting in a chair at the office in a (**63**) _____. It is also a slightly hereditary complaint.

This is by no means the same as the night-time cramp already mentioned, and there is no absolute cure. The patient learns to (**64**) _____ the amount of exercise he or she can comfortably take.

No drugs offer a complete relief but there is one habit which the sufferer must (**65**) _____—smoking. Whatever may or may not be one's views about the habit, it undoubtedly makes intermittent claudication far more troublesome.

A number of patients will secretly admit that so long as they keep off tobacco they do not get this fearsome cramp.

56. **A.** strenuous   **B.** working   **C.** painful   **D.** relaxed

57. **A.** doing   **B.** avoiding   **C.** taking   **D.** changing

58. **A.** dizzy   **B.** lazy   **C.** crazy   **D.** fuzzy

59. **A.** important   **B.** interesting   **C.** serious   **D.** dangerous

60. **A.** complex   **B.** difficult   **C.** likely   **D.** pronounced

61. **A.** speak   **B.** continue   **C.** stand   **D.** act

62. **A.** impressed   **B.** affected   **C.** emphasized   **D.** learned

63. **A.** draught   **B.** drought   **C.** draughts   **D.** droughts

64. **A.** rule   **B.** regulate   **C.** take   **D.** understand

65. **A.** give out   **B.** give back   **C.** give away   **D.** give up

Ⅲ   Writing

 Question 66

- Write about medical reform in China.
  Medical reform has been an issue that affects residents' livelihood. Please briefly analyze the current problems in health care system and give your own advice on medical reform.
- Write an essay of no less than 150 words on your answer sheet.

医护英语水平考试（三级）

模拟训练（七）

Medical English Test System（METS）
Level 3

Ⅰ　Listening

Part One　>>>>>>

 Questions 1—5

- You will hear five extracts from conversations taking place in different clinical departments.
- Choose which case each doctor is discussing from the list **A—F**.
- Use each letter **A—F** only once. There is one extra letter which you **DO NOT** need to use.
- Mark the corresponding letter on your **answer sheet**.
- You will hear each extract twice.

Doctor 1   **1**

Doctor 2   **2**

Doctor 3   **3**

Doctor 4   **4**

Doctor 5   **5**

A. The patient is allowed to leave the hospital.

B. The patient is going to receive a CT.

C. The patient is diagnosed with pneumonia and neuroleptic malignant syndrome.

D. The patient has to take insulin.

E. The patient has some problem with the eyes.

F. The patient is easily fractured.

Part Two >>>>>>

 ### Questions 6—13

- You will hear a conversation between a reporter and a hair restoration expert.
- For each of the following statements, decide whether it is **True (A)** or **False (B)**. If there is not enough information to answer **True (A)** or **False (B)**, choose **Not Given (C)**.
- Mark the corresponding letter on your **answer sheet**.
- You will hear the recording twice.

---

6. Hair loss is a part of the normal aging process for most women.
   A. True   **B.** False   **C.** Not Given

7. Some types of female hair loss are due to hormone changes.
   A. True   **B.** False   **C.** Not Given

8. Women may experience hair loss after giving birth.
   A. True   **B.** False   **C.** Not Given

9. Men tend to see hair loss start at the temples.
   A. True   **B.** False   **C.** Not Given

10. It is necessary to see a doctor for sudden hair loss.
    A. True   **B.** False   **C.** Not Given

11. Minoxidil is an over-the-counter drug.
    A. True   **B.** False   **C.** Not Given

12. Hair transplantation is not a good choice for women.
    A. True   **B.** False   **C.** Not Given

13. New hair growth occurs in as little as two months.
    A. True   **B.** False   **C.** Not Given

Part Three >>>>>>

 ### Questions 14—20

- You will hear a discussion among an instructor and two medical students.
- For questions **14—20**, choose the most appropriate answer.
- Mark the corresponding letter on your **answer sheet**.
- You will hear the discussion twice.

14. Efforts with gene therapy for brain cancer were largely limited because _____.

    A. the drug could not be delivered into the brain

    B. the drug was not fully effective

    C. the drug had some side-effects

15. What prevents drugs from reaching the cancer cells in brain tumor patients?

    A. The blood-brain block.

    B. The blood-brain barrier.

    C. The blood-brain defense.

16. In the new treatment，the blood brain barrier is by-passed by _____.

    A. directly injecting the chemotherapy into the region of the tumor

    B. directly injecting the gene therapy into the region of the tumor

    C. directly injecting the drugs into the region of the tumor

17. The MRI-guided process provides _____ confirmation that adequate amount of the therapy is delivered into the tumor.

    A. acoustic   **B.** tactile   **C.** visual

18. Which of the following therapy is based on a retrovirus engineered to selectively replicate in high grade brain cancer cells?

    A. The gene therapy.

    B. The chemotherapy.

    C. The hydrotherapy.

19. When chemotherapy is given，how many cells in the body are exposed to the potential side-effects of the drug?

    A. Almost all the cells.

    B. Nearly half of the cells in the body.

    D. It depends on the type of chemotherapy.

20. What are the risks of the new treatment?

    A. The retrovirus.

    B. The unintended injury.

    C. The surgical procedure itself.

Part Four　>>>>>>

Questions 21—25

- You will hear a speech on diets helping some people with Hashimoto's disease.
- Complete the notes. In each blank，write only one word.

- Write the answers on your **answer sheet**.
- You will hear the speech twice.

Notes:

- Hashimoto's disease is the most common autoimmune condition and the leading cause of (**21**) _____.

  The thyroid gland plays a major role in metabolism, hormone regulation, and body temperature.

There are different diets that can help people with Hashimoto's disease:

- Gluten-free diets remove all foods with containing gluten, which is a (**22**) _____ found in wheat, barley, rye, and other grains.

  There is no current research to support a gluten-free diet for all people with Hashimoto's.

- A grain-free diet is very similar to gluten-free, except that grains are also off-limits.

- The paleo diet emphasizes on whole and (**23**) _____ foods.

- People who do not want to focus on what foods to cut out can choose a nutrient-dense diet.

  Having foods such as colorful fruits will leave less room for processed and refined sugar foods.

  (**24**) _____ spices such as turmeric are also encouraged.

- It is more important for a person to follow a (**25**) _____ diet.

  People with Hashimoto's should try different eating styles and find the best one for them.

Ⅱ Reading

Part One >>>>>>

 Questions 26—35

• Read the following passage about low-salt diet.

Scientists Advise: Low-Salt Diet Not for Everyone

1 Low-salt diets are actually harmful to our bodies, a recent study found. These diets may actually increase the risk of developing heart disease, or even cause death. These findings, says WebMD, a public health website, are contrary to the popular wisdom that has long said low-salt diets are healthy.

2 Scientists at McMaster University's Population Health Research Institute, working with researchers from Hamilton Health Services, conducted the study. They examined medical information about 130,000 people from 49 countries. The scientists, led by Andrew Mente of McMaster University, wanted to find out if the relationship between salt, strokes and heart disease is different for those who have high blood pressure. They found that no matter whether one has high blood pressure or not, low sodium intake increased the risk of stroke, heart attack and death. The study goes on to suggest that only certain people should be concerned about reducing sodium in their diets. "The findings emphasize the importance of reducing salt intake among people with hypertension and who eat food with high levels of sodium," Mente said.

3 McMaster University's Martin O'Donnell, the study's co-author, said in a press release in May 2016, "This study adds to our understanding of the relationship between salt intake and health. The study also questions the correctness of present guidelines that recommend low salt intake for everyone." He noted, "An approach that recommends salt in moderation, particularly focused on those with hypertension, appears more in-line with current evidence." Mente added that the current general recommendations relating to the maximum healthy salt intake seems too low, especially since they do not consider an individual's blood pressure. "One of those effects includes harmful elevation of particular hormones—and this offsets any benefits. The main issue is not whether very low sodium intake lowers blood pressure, but whether it results in improved health," Mente said.

4 In the McMaster University study, the researchers found that only around 10% of people had high levels of both hypertension and sodium consumption. In general, health experts consider a high level of sodium consumption to be over 6 grams daily. Mente pointed out that this indicates that many people around the world are taking in healthy amounts of salt. He also said that efforts should be targeted at reducing salt intake among the people who are most likely to get hypertension and who take in high amounts of salt. Mente does not agree with the current strategy of reducing sodium intake in almost all countries.

5   At present, Canadians normally consume about 4 grams of sodium daily. But there are recommendations that they should lower this amount to less than 2.3 grams each day. US guidelines for sodium intake are for people under 50 to have less than 2.3 grams a day. For those over 51 and persons of any age who are African American or have hypertension, diabetes, or chronic kidney disease, the US guidelines suggest having less than 1.5 grams a day. In Kenya, the Ministry of Public Health and Sanitation recommends general reduction of salt intake to levels below 5 grams as recommended by the World Health Organization. This is as a measure to reduce the risk of hypertension and other non-communicable diseases. Less than 5% of people in the world consume such low levels of sodium. Kenyans are the lowest consumers of salt, averaging 4 grams a day.

 ## Questions 26—30

- Choose the most appropriate subheading from the list **A—F** for each paragraph.
- Use each letter **A—F** only once. There is one extra letter which you **DO NOT** need to use.
- Mark the corresponding letter on your **answer sheet**.

26. Paragraph 1 _____

27. Paragraph 2 _____

28. Paragraph 3 _____

29. Paragraph 4 _____

30. Paragraph 5 _____

> **A.** Brief description of purpose, methods, results and suggestions of the study.
> **B.** Most people taking in healthy amounts of salt while level of sodium consumption for some people depending on their health conditions.
> **C.** Proposing the idea of low-salt diets being harmful to human bodies.
> **D.** Examples of recommendations for correct sodium intake daily in different countries.
> **E.** Some doubts about current recommendations for healthy salt intake.
> **F.** Researchers recommending people to have the same sodium intake in almost all countries.

Questions 31—35

- Fill in each blank with the correct answer from the list **A—F**.
- Use each letter **A—F** only once. There is one extra letter which you **DO NOT** need to use.
- Mark the corresponding letter on your **answer sheet**.

31. WebMD points out that these findings are _____ the popular wisdom that low-salt diets are good for health for a long time.

32. The study continues to advise that only some people should be worried about _____ in their diets.

33. The research also doubts the correctness of _____ , which suggests low salt intake for everyone.

34. Mente disagrees with the _____ of cutting down sodium intake in almost all countries.

35. The U. S. guidelines recommend having less than one point five grams per day for those who have hypertension, diabetes, or chronic _____ .

> **A.** kidney disease
> **B.** present guidelines
> **C.** sodium consumption
> **D.** reducing sodium
> **E.** contrary to
> **F.** current strategy

Part Two >>>>>>

Questions 36—42

- Read the following passage about patient history.
- Choose the best answer **A, B, C** or **D**.
- Mark the corresponding letter on your **answer sheet**.

The Patient History

A detailed patient history and physical exam form the foundation of patient evaluation and vital patient data that enable efficient, quality patient rounds. On the other hand, a poorly documented history and physical exam may lead to confusion, serious omission of vital data and inefficiency on patient rounds.

The basic outline structure for the patient history and physical exam usually includes the following:

Identification: patient name, age, gender, race, and occupation

Chief Complaint: (in the patient's words)

HPI: (history of present illness)

PMHx: (past medical history)

ROS: review of systems

Social Hx: includes family situation(married, divorced, single), habits, cigarettes, alcohol or illicit drug use, sexual behavior

Here are a few specific points about each section of the history outline:

Identification—This should include the patient's name, age, sex, race and occupation. For example: "Mr. Jones is a 55-year-old Caucasian male who works as a farmer." The patient's name written in the history allows future interviewers to address the patient by his name which conveys a sense of patient respect. The age, race, sex and occupation are important as many diseases are not only gender and age dependent, but may also occur more commonly in specific ethnic and occupation groups.

Chief Complaint—This should be written in the patient's words. For example, "chest pain" rather than "angina". Also the duration of the chief complaint should be noted "chest pain for 1 hour". Before moving on to the HPI, it would be appropriate to perform a "survey of problems" asking the patient if there are any other current problems bothering them.

HPI (History of Present Illness)—The history of the present illness is a more elaborate description of the patient's chief complaint and is the most important structural element of the medical history. This section should give the following details about the chief complaint (s):

a. Detailed description of the "chief complaint"; "a dull crushing chest pain" including body location of the complaint.

b. A chronological history and sequence of the chief complaint.

c. What circumstances precipitate it: climbing stairs, emotional upset such as anger, or sexual intercourse.

d. What circumstances relieve it: resting for a few minutes.

ROS (Review of Systems)—This section is too often omitted. Although it is somewhat cumbersome to go through a "complete" review of systems and it may not be necessary to do so for "each" admission, at least one "complete" review of systems should be documented in the patient's medical record. For subsequent admissions, the history could simply refer back to the "complete ROS" documented on a specified date.

Social History—This section is the most neglected section of the patient history performed in China. Vital information such as smoking history, use of alcohol or illicit drugs and sexual behavior can give invaluable clues to the diagnosis. Also documentation of the patient's marital status (divorced) and family situation may give clues to the early diagnosis of anxiety or depression.

In summary，the patient history is the most important aspect of patient evaluation as it guides the physician team's decisions concerning diagnostic workup and formulation of a treatment plan. As mentioned the patient history contributes more towards the diagnosis than any other test. Further it can help to establish rapport where the patient not only learns to trust his/her physician but also is more likely to heed his/her advice.

36. According to the author，a poorly documented history and physical exam may cause the following results EXCEPT _____.
    A. a lack of efficiency
    B. negligence of important data
    C. the situation of being confused
    D. misdiagnosis

37. Why is Identification considered an important part of the patient history?
    A. They convey a sense of patient respect.
    B. A lot of diseases are gender and age dependent.
    C. Many diseases occur more commonly in specific ethnic and occupation groups.
    D. All the above answers are correct.

38. According to the passage，which of the following is NOT the basic outline structure for the patient history and physical exam?
    A. Patient's history of present and past sickness.
    B. Statement of sickness should be written in patient's words.
    C. Treatment plan.
    D. Patient's profession, gender, sexual behavior, and illegal drug use.

39. Which of the following statement is true?
    A. Chief complaint should be written according to the doctor's experience.
    B. In the course of the chief complaint，it would be proper to ask patients a "survey of problems" possibly bothering them.
    C. HPI gives a more detailed presentation of the patient's chief complaint.
    D. HPI should present what circumstances precipitate illness and relieve illness.

40. According to the passage, what is NOT true about ROS and Social History?
    A. At least one integral review of systems should be recorded.
    B. ROS and Social History are the most omitted section of the patient history performed in China.
    C. Social History can give very useful clues to the diagnosis.
    D. The early diagnosis of anxiety or depression may be seen in the patient's marital status and family situation.

41. What does the underlined word "rapport" probably mean?

    A. Good relationship.

    B. Effective communication.

    C. Favorable environment.

    D. Well-deserved reputation.

42. The author's purpose in writing this passage is _____.

    A. to introduce the basic structure of the patient history

    B. to introduce negative effects of a poorly documented patient history

    C. to emphasize the importance of the patient history

    D. to present how the patient history affects a treatment plan

Part Three >>>>>>

 ## Questions 43—50

- Read the following passage about a coffee cancer warning.
- For each of the following statements, decide whether it is **True (A)** or **False (B)**. If there is not enough information to answer **True (A)** or **False (B)**, choose **Not Given (C)**.
- Mark the corresponding letter on your **answer sheet**.

Coffee Cancer Warning: What Science Says about the Actual Risk

Trouble is brewing for coffee lovers in California, where a judge ruled that sellers must post scary warnings about cancer risks. But how frightened should we be of a daily cup of coffee? Not very, some scientists and available evidence seem to suggest.

Scientific concerns about coffee have eased in recent years, and many studies even suggest it can help health. "At the minimum, coffee is neutral. If anything, there is fairly good evidence of the benefit of coffee on cancer," said Dr. Edward Giovannucci, a nutrition expert at the Harvard School of Public Health.

CBS News medical contributor Dr. David Agus, director of the Westside Cancer Center at USC, says he believes it is too early to put this kind of blanket warning on coffee.

"When you put a bold declaration that 'X may cause cancer' when there isn't data to that effect in humans, to me it causes panic rather than informed knowledge," he told *CBS This Morning*.

The World Health Organization's cancer agency moved coffee off the "possible carcinogen" list two years ago, though it says evidence is insufficient to rule out any possible role.

The current flap isn't about coffee itself, but a chemical called acrylamide that's made when the beans are roasted. Government agencies call it a probable or likely carcinogen, based on animal research, and a group sued to require coffee sellers to warn of that under a California law passed by voters in 1986.

Coffee and your health

The problem: No one knows what levels are safe or risky for people. The US Environmental Protection Agency sets acrylamide limits for drinking water, but there aren't any for food.

"A cup of coffee a day, exposure probably is not that high," and probably should not change your habit, said Dr. Bruce Y. Lee of Johns Hopkins Bloomberg School of Public Health. "If you drink a lot of cups a day, this is one of the reasons you might consider cutting that down."

The chemical

Start with the biggest known risk factor for cancer—smoking—which generates acrylamide. In the diet, French fries, potato chips, crackers, cookies, cereal and other high-carbohydrate foods contain it as a byproduct of roasting, baking, toasting or frying.

What's the risk?

The "probable" or "likely" carcinogen label is based on studies of animals given high levels of acrylamide in drinking water. But people and rodents absorb the chemical at different rates and metabolize it differently, so its relevance to human health is unknown.

A group of 23 scientists convened by the WHO's cancer agency in 2016 looked at coffee—not acrylamide directly—and decided coffee was unlikely to cause breast, prostate or pancreatic cancer, and that it seemed to lower the risks for liver and uterine cancers. Evidence was inadequate to determine its effect on dozens of other cancer types.

43. According to some available evidence, we are not very afraid of cancer risks that coffee may cause.

    A. True   **B.** False   **C.** Not Given

44. Many studies even show that coffee can help health, and scientific worries about coffee have decreased in recent years.

    A. True   **B.** False   **C.** Not Given

45. There is a concern that the warning label may cause panic instead of informed knowledge.

    A. True   **B.** False   **C.** Not Given

46. The World Health Organization has made a plan to prevent possible risk of cancer.

    A. True   **B.** False   **C.** Not Given

47. Government agencies are sure that a chemical called acrylamide is a carcinogen.

    A. True   **B.** False   **C.** Not Given

48. According to Dr. Bruce Y. Lee, drinking coffee should be moderate.

    A. True   **B.** False   **C.** Not Given

49. Smoking which is harmful to health can cause lung cancer.

    A. True   **B.** False   **C.** Not Given

50. In 2016, the WHO's cancer agency convened a group of 23 scientists, who considered coffee had a high risk of causing breast, prostate or pancreatic cancer.

    A. True   **B.** False   **C.** Not Given

Part Four >>>>>>

 Questions 51—55

- Read the following passage about the pills. Five sentences have been removed from the passage.
- Fill in each blank with the most appropriate sentence from the list **A—F**. There is one extra sentence which you **DO NOT** need to use.
- Mark the corresponding letter on your **answer sheet.**

The Pills

These days there are pills for just about everything. If you can't sleep, take a pill. If you're sad, take a pill. If you're in pain, take a pill. But what about people who are overweight or lack fitness? **(51)** _____ Drug companies are always looking for new pills to sell, and many have spent lots of money on developing a pill for these people too. In the 1990s, scientists working for one of these companies found a new drug that gave mice some of the same benefits as exercise. Newspapers began reporting on this new drug, calling it the "fitness pill" or "exercise pill".

The reports said that mice with no previous fitness training could run much longer distances after being given the drug. They said there was evidence that the drug could also help humans by improving fitness and building up muscles. Many people who read these articles wanted to try the pills, but reports about problems with the drug soon began appearing. **(52)** _____ This meant the drug would never be approved for human use and the drug company stopped developing it.

Medical researchers are still looking for a drug similar to the one found in the 90s. **(53)** _____ They believe such a drug would have many uses, including important medical uses. It could benefit people who can't get out of bed due to ill health. It could also benefit people with diabetes and those with diseases that cause muscle-wasting. **(54)** _____ Most adults say they don't have enough spare time to do the 40 minutes of daily exercise that doctors recommend. For these people, a so-called fitness pill or exercise pill could be the best solution. But others might say they're cheating by taking a pill instead of exercising. Would you take such a pill if it meant you no longer had to jog, swim or use a treadmill to stay fit?

(55) _____ They fear that some athletes might use it as a performance-enhancing drug. Even though the drug discovered in the 90s was never approved for human use, some athletes may have used it to cheat. Top athletes already go through extensive drug testing before national and international events, but until sports authorities know about a new drug, it won't be tested for. Some people think top athletes who pass drug tests might still be cheating, and in some cases this has been shown to be true. The world-famous swimmer and Olympic gold-medalist Michael Phelps knew this, so he offered to go through extra drug testing before the 2008 Olympics. He knew that many people would suspect his amazing strength and stamina came from using performance-enhancing drugs, so he felt he had to prove that it came from hard work and training alone.

A. Medical researchers also believe such a drug could benefit the average adult as well.

B. They're trying to find a new drug with the same benefits that doesn't also cause cancer.

C. They said it could "build muscle, increase stamina, and even burn fat."

D. The best solution for these people is to exercise, but many people don't want to exercise or are unable to exercise.

E. Researchers found that mice had an increased chance of developing cancer after taking it.

F. Many people in the world of sports are concerned about a pill like this.

Part Five >>>>>

 ## Questions 56—65

- Read the following passage about a study of weight.
- Fill in each blank with the correct choice **A**, **B**, **C** or **D**.
- Mark the corresponding letter on your **answer sheet**.

Study: Nearly a Third of World Overweight

A new study finds one third of the world's population is overweight or considered obese. Since 1980, obesity rates in children and adults have doubled in 73 countries. And rates are increasing in many other countries, according to a report released on Monday.

The report was published in the *New England Journal of Medicine*.

Obesity is increasing faster in children than adults in many nations, including Algeria, Turkey and Jordan, the report said. But the world's weight problem is (**56**) _____ in both rich and poor countries alike.

Researchers say an increasing number of people are dying of (**57**) _____ health problems in what they called a "disturbing global public health crisis."

About four million people died of cardiovascular disease, diabetes, cancer and other diseases linked to (**58**) _____ weight in 2015, according to the study.

"People who shrug off weight gain do so at their own risk," said Christopher Murray, one of the writers of the report.

Researchers studied health information from 1980 through 2015. They (**59**) _____ obesity rates, average weight gain and the cause of death in 195 countries. They found that obesity rates are three times greater among youth and young adults in countries like China, Brazil and India.

Almost 108 million children and more than 600 million adults were found to be obese. Together, that represents about 10 percent of the world's population.

Among the top 20 most (**60**) _____ countries in 2015, Egypt had the highest number of age-standardized obese adults. Vietnam had the least. In the same year, the United States had the highest number of obese children, and Bangladesh had the least.

Researchers say the extra weight people are carrying increases their risk of (**61**) _____ diabetes or other health problems.

(**62**) _____ hunger remains a problem in many areas. The United Nations estimates that almost 800 million people, including 300 million children, go to bed hungry each night.

Experts said poor diets and lack of physical activity are mainly to (**63**) _____ for the rising numbers of overweight people.

Growing populations have (**64**) _____ rising obesity rates in poor countries. Often, poor people will eat processed foods instead of choosing a diet rich in vegetables.

"People are consuming more and more processed foods that are high in sugar and fat and exercising less," said Boitshepo Giyose, senior nutrition officer at the UN Food and Agriculture Organization.

The London-based Overseas Development Institute studied the price of food in five countries: Britain, Brazil, China, Mexico and South Korea. It found that the cost of processed foods like ice cream and hamburgers has (**65**) _____ since 1990. But the cost of fresh fruits and vegetables has gone up.

56. **A.** decreasing **B.** growing **C.** falling **D.** changing

57. **A.** related **B.** big **C.** complex **D.** annoying

58. **A.** extra **B.** extensive **C.** excess **D.** undue

59. A. saw   **B.** read   **C.** tested   **D.** examined

60. A. populous   **B.** developed   **C.** developing   **D.** vulnerable

61. A. gaining   **B.** acquiring   **C.** getting   **D.** developing

62. A. And   **B.** So   **C.** Yet   **D.** Though

63. A. blame   **B.** scold   **C.** condemn   **D.** charge

64. A. resulted from   **B.** brought about   **C.** attributed to   **D.** given out

65. A. risen   **B.** climbed   **C.** fallen   **D.** surged

Ⅲ Writing

 Question 66

- Write about the following topic.

  Some people believe that the best way to lead a healthy life is doing regular exercises, while others assert that emotional management is of greater importance. What do you think?

- Write an essay of no less than 150 words on your answer sheet.

听力文本、参考答案及解析

医护英语水平考试(三级)
模拟训练(一)

听力文本

This is METS-3 listening test. There are four parts in the test, Part One, Two, Three, and Four. You will hear each part twice. We will now stop for a moment before we start the test. Please ask any questions because you must not speak during the test. Now, look at the instructions for Part One.

You will hear five extracts from conversations taking place in different clinical departments. Choose which case each doctor is discussing from the list A—F. Use each letter A—F only once. There is one extra letter which you do not need to use. Mark the corresponding letter on your answer sheet. You will hear each extract twice. Now we are ready to start.

Extract 1

You'll receive an intravenous injection. Make a tight fist. Now open it. This injection contains the medicine which can be seen by the machine so that it is possible for us to scan your kidney. You have to wait so that the medicine can reach your kidney. You must not move during the scan. We'll send the results to your doctor.

Extract 2

We are going to do a scan of the brain called CT scan or CAT scan. This is an easy test. You just need to lie on a special stretcher which moves and runs into the head scanner. It's a little bit like putting your head in a large washing machine. You lie still and you will hear the machine making noises while it takes some special cross-sectional X-rays to give us a picture of your brain.

Extract 3

I am sorry to have to tell you that you do have an eye tumor and we'll have to do something about it. I'm afraid that it's melanoma of the eye. It's in an advanced stage so it is very likely that we will have to remove the eye itself. I know that sounds very drastic but eye tumors behave differently from other tumors in the body so there's a high chance that once we take the eye out, that will be the end of the tumor and the cancer will be removed totally.

Extract 4

Mr. Brown, open your eyes. The operation is over. Take deep breaths. Give us a cough. I'm going to clean your mouth. Open your mouth wide. Spit out what you have in your mouth. It's time to wake up. Can you breathe? How is your breathing? I'm going to take the tube out of your mouth. Do you feel sick? Are you in any pain? We are going to transfer you to the recovery room.

Extract 5

Well, while I'm feeling his stomach, I can feel a little lump underneath my fingers and what indicates to me is that he's got some overgrowth of the muscle at the exit of the stomach, and that's blocking the material like milk draining from his stomach. So I think it's likely that what we need to do is a small operation to cut through the muscle and relax it.

Now you'll hear Part One again. This is the end of Part One. Now look at Part Two. You will hear a conversation between two doctors. For each of the following statements, decide whether it is True (A) or False (B). If there is not enough information to answer True (A) or False (B), choose Not Given (C). Mark the corresponding letter on your answer sheet. You will hear the recording twice.

Doctor A: Hello, Jim. I wonder if you could see a patient for me.

Doctor B: Certainly, Mary. What's the story?

Doctor A: Well, it's Mr. Alan Jameson, a 53-year-old carpenter. He had been an infrequent attender but he came to see me this morning complaining of pain in his right leg and his back.

Doctor B: And when did this start?

Doctor A: Well, it came on about six weeks ago and it's become gradually more severe over the past couple of weeks.

Doctor B: Was the pain localized?

Doctor A: No. At first he thought he'd just pulled a muscle. But it's got so bad that he hasn't been able to do his work properly. It's also been getting to the stage where the pain is waking him up at night. It's been so severe. He's also noticed some tingling in his right foot. He's having difficulty in carrying on with his work. He's also lost three kilos and become quite depressed.

Doctor B: Did he have any similar symptoms in the past?

Doctor A: No, not exactly, but he has suffered from intermittent pain in the back. Paracetamol gave some relief but didn't solve the problem completely.

Doctor B: Apart from that, any other problems with health in the past?

Doctor A: No, perfectly OK.

Doctor B: Did you find anything else on examination?

Doctor A: Yes, as well as the pain he has numbness in his toes on the right foot.

Now you'll hear Part Two again. This is the end of Part Two. Now look at Part Three. You will hear a discussion among a supervising physician and two medical students. For questions 14—20, choose the most appropriate answer. Mark the corresponding letter on your answer sheet. You will hear the discussion twice.

Supervising physician: Today I'll explain acute severe asthma. Do you have any questions?

Student 1: I've learned that asthma is prevalent in modern society.

Supervising physician: Yes, it strikes a surprisingly large number of Americans.

Student 2: What is the cause of asthma?

Supervising physician: The actual triggers of asthma are varied, but some of the common ones are cold air, exercise, infection, common viruses, irritants and allergies.

Student 1: Does genetics play a role in asthma?

Supervising physician: Several studies show that heredity will increase the chances of developing asthma. But one will not definitely develop it because of heredity.

Student 2: Is it serious?

Supervising physician: Yes, it can cause death. Approximately 5,000 people die of asthma every year.

Student 2: Could you tell us what happens in an asthma attack?

Supervising physician: What have you learned about it?

Student 1: I think there are three components.

Supervising physician: Yes, you are right. It is usually thought to involve three components: swelling of the airways, constriction of the muscles around the airways, and inflammation.

Student 1: How about acute severe asthma?

Supervising physician: It is also called status asthmatics, and it is an attack of severe bronchospasm that is unresponsive to routine therapy.

Student 1: What are the characteristics of acute severe asthma?

Supervising physician: The attack may be sudden and may be rapidly fatal, often before

	medical care can be obtained.
Student 2:	Can you tell us the symptoms of acute severe asthma?
Supervising physician:	Patients will have difficulty in talking, and they use accessory muscles of inspiration, and they will have orthopnea.
Student 1:	How should we deal with this problem?
Supervising physician:	The treatment should be immediate and aggressive.
Student 2:	Do we have to monitor blood oxygen saturation?
Supervising physician:	Yes, at the same time there should be arterial blood gas analysis to evaluate hypercarbia. And we should measure frequently the peak expiratory flow rate.
Student 1:	What special attention should we pay to these patients?
Supervising physician:	These patients require continuous direct observation and monitoring.
Student 1:	That means the patients should be closely watched?
Supervising physician:	Yes, it is one kind of emergency case.
Student 1:	We've got it. Thank you.

Now you'll hear Part Three again. This is the end of Part Three. Now look at Part Four. You will hear a speech on various contraceptive methods. Complete the notes. In each blank, write only one word. Write the answers on your answer sheet. You will hear the speech twice.

Female: There are different types of contraceptive pills that you need to think about and they all work differently. There's what we call the mini-pill which has a single hormone in it but you do need to be more careful about when you take it because it only has a three-hour gap in which it is safe and if you take it any later than that, then it's not working reliably.

The combined pill on the other hand has two types of hormones in it, and it has a much wider range. You can be up to 12 hours late and it'll still work reliably. However some people do find that they have problems with both types of pills, for example, they get headaches or migraines or put on weight and some people also have problems with their blood pressure, so it is not always suitable.

Another option is to have a coil; however, we don't normally recommend this to women until they've had at least one child, because some studies have shown that although the coil isn't necessarily associated with causing infections, if you do have any pelvic inflammatory diseases, it can be made worse, and it can increase the risk of infertility. Therefore, it is usually only given to women after they've had at least one child.

The cap or diaphragm has its advantages in that it doesn't involve any hormones, therefore, you're not messing around with your body's cycle and it also means that it can be put in before you have your intercourse not like the sheath or anything so it's in and out of the way and out of your mind. However, you do have to have it quite carefully fitted and you need to be quite confident with your own body in learning how to put it in. If you are at all embarrassed, it can be very difficult.

If you are absolutely certain that you've finished your family or you're not planning on having any children, it's possible to be sterilized or as it is sometimes called "have your tubes tied". This normally involves just a minor operation. You are just in for a day. We look inside your stomach with a telescope and cut and tie off each of your tubes to stop the egg from reaching the womb, and it stops you from getting pregnant. It's a very, very reliable method. It has a very low failure rate, but its main drawback is that it should be regarded as being absolutely irreversible, and once it's done you really can't have it changed back. So you have to be very sure that you don't want any more children.

Coitus interruptus, also called the rhythm method, is a very unreliable method of contraception, where the man withdraws from the female just before he comes. However, there is often a small quantity of sperm released even before the man comes, and, therefore, it's an extremely unreliable method.

Condoms or sheaths are quite a safe and reliable method of contraception. The main disadvantage is that they have to be put on during or shortly before intercourse, and this can, therefore, interrupt the spontaneity of lovemaking. However, they do have the advantage of protecting against sexually transmitted diseases.

Now you'll hear Part Four again. This is the end of Part Four. You now have five minutes to write your answers on the answer sheet. You have one more minute. This is the end of the listening test.

参考答案与试题评析

I Listening
Part One
1.【语段大意】医生正对患者解释静脉内肾盂造影(intravenous pyelogram)。在此过程中,患者先握拳,再松开,进行静脉造影剂的注射,使注射液含有的造影物质慢慢到达肾部,便于扫描。

【解题思路】F 可听到 intravenous injection, scan your kidney, can reach your kidney 等关键信息。

2.【语段大意】医生正对患者解释脑部 CT 扫描术(brain CT)。在此过程中,患者躺在

5

特殊担架上(a special stretcher)被送入头部扫描仪(head scanner),保持不动,直到机器发出声音,照下脑部的断层扫描 X 片。

【解题思路】B 可听到 a scan of the brain called CT scan or CAT scan, head scanner, your head, a picture of your brain 等关键信息。

3.【语段大意】患者疑患有眼部黑素瘤(melanoma of the eye),已晚期(in an advanced stage)。医生可能会采取眼球切除(remove the eye)的方法,并向患者解释采取此措施的原因在于眼部肿瘤不同于其他区域的肿瘤,可通过眼球切除,彻底根除。

【解题思路】A 可听到 an eye tumor, the eye, eye tumors, take the eye out 等关键词。

4.【语段大意】患者刚接受完手术,医生试图通过引导患者深呼吸、咳嗽、清洗口腔等一系列动作来检查患者的意识状态,接着送患者至恢复室(recovery room)。

【解题思路】D 可听到 The operation is over. 这一关键句。

5.【语段大意】本题描述的是一名正在接受医生体检的患者,医生通过指检,触摸到指下胃部硬块(a little lump underneath my fingers),疑为胃出口处肌肉增生(overgrowth of the muscle at the exit of the stomach),计划采取手术来治疗(cut through the muscle and relax it)。

【解题思路】E 可听到 his stomach, the stomach, from his stomach 等关键信息。

Part Two
【语篇大意】两位医生针对患者病情的讨论。
【解题思路】

6. B 对话开头就提到医生 Jim 非常乐意替 Mary 看看她患者的情况,故答案为 B。

7. B 对话中 Mary 提及过去多年患者 Alan Jameson 很少来看病(infrequent attender),故答案为 B。

8. A 当 Jim 问到疾病发作时间时,Mary 提到约六周前开始(about six weeks ago),所以答案为 A。

9. A 起初病人以为是肌肉拉伤,但后来疼痛非常严重,以至于难以正常工作,夜间都会被疼痛折磨醒,所以 A 正确。

10. B 患者体重下降三公斤,精神抑郁,因此选 B。

11. B 患者提及疼痛非常严重,在右足处可感到刺痛(tingling),而并非在右手处,所以选 B。

12. B 患者之前曾在背部出现间歇性疼痛(intermittent pain),用药也未见治愈,所以选 B。

13. C 整篇对话并未提及患者诊断结果,故 C 正确。

Part Three
【语篇大意】两位医学生向临床老师咨询哮喘的相关问题。
【解题思路】

14. A 对话中提及哮喘诱因各不相同,但通常有冷空气、运动、感染、常见病毒、刺激物及过敏。本题 B 与 C 均对,故 A 为答案。关键信息:What is the cause of asthma? /The actual triggers of asthma are varied, but some of the common ones are cold air, exercise, infection, common viruses, irritants and allergies.

15. C 对话中提到研究表明遗传会增加哮喘的发病率,而非性格与饮食,故答案为 C。

关键信息：Several studies show that heredity will increase the chances of developing asthma. But one will not definitely develop it because of heredity.

16. B 对话中提到哮喘会致死,每年大约 5 000 人死于哮喘,所以答案应该选 B。关键信息：Yes, it can cause death. Approximately 5 000 people die of asthma every year.

17. B 对话中提到哮喘发作有三个方面组成:气道水肿（swelling of the airways）,气道周围肌肉收缩（constriction of the muscles around the airways)及炎症。选项 A 和 C 均对,B 选项的全身肌肉收缩,不符,故答案为 B。关键信息：three components：swelling of the airways, constriction of the muscles around the airways, and inflammation.

18. C 关于急性严重哮喘(acute severe asthma)的发作,对话中提到它是一种严重支气管痉挛(bronchospasm),对常规治疗无效,故 A 不符;它发作迅速,通常致命,故 B 不符;症状包括谈话困难与端坐呼吸(orthopnea),显然 C 正确。关键信息：Can you tell us the symptoms of acute severe asthma? /Patients will have difficulty in talking, and they use accessory muscles of inspiration, and they will have orthopnea.

19. A 对话中提到急性严重哮喘（acute severe asthma）的治疗应该迅速、积极(immediate and aggressive),故答案为 A。关键信息：The treatment should be immediate and aggressive.

20. A 对话中提到对哮喘患者应进行血氧饱和度监控(monitor blood oxygen saturation),同时进行动脉血气分析(arterial blood gas analysis),防止出现高碳酸血症(hypercarbia）等,故答案为 A。关键信息：Do we have to monitor blood oxygen saturation? /Yes, at the same time there should be arterial blood gas analysis to evaluate hypercarbia.

Part Four
【语篇大意】关于不同避孕方式利弊的一段讲座。
【解题思路】

21. mini-pill 此处为讲座中提到的第一个避孕方式,即为一种含有单个激素的小剂量避孕药片,因其仅房事前后三个小时有效,所以使用需特别小心。所以此处应填 mini-pill。

22. migraines 文中讲述前两种避孕药使用时会出现头痛（headaches）、偏头痛(migraines)、体重增加、血压问题等副作用。所以此处应填 migraines。

23. infertility 文章建议已育女性使用宫内避孕环(coil),并且说明其副作用为加重盆腔炎(pelvic inflammatory diseases)的程度,及增加不孕症(infertility)风险。根据短文内容,此处应填 infertility。

24. irreversible 文中讲述到输卵管结扎手术时,提到其主要缺点为手术的不可逆性(irreversible),故此处应填 irreversible。

25. sexually 文中提到避孕套这种避孕方式时,提到其主要优点即为防止性传播疾病(sexually transmitted diseases)。故此处应填 sexually。

Ⅱ Reading
Part One
【文章大意】文章指出良好的饮食习惯与持之以恒的体育运动是健康的保证,并给出了一些营养饮食的建议。

【解题思路】

26. A 根据第一段第一句"Making wise food choices early in life will help prevent health problems that can effect you later."和最后一句"Your eating habits ... are crucial elements on the path to a healthier body and self.",合理饮食是保持健康的不二选择;第二句"It is reported that 8 of the 10 leading causes of death in America are directly related to what we eat and drink."则是对这一主题的反面论证。

27. B 第二段段首提出应限制脂肪的摄入"Experts recommend limiting your fat intake to 30% of the total calories you consume per day.",段中指出减肥应该少食多动"If you want to lose weight ... eat less and exercise more.",而段末又提及过度节食伤及身体"Starvation diets or losing weight too fast can be dangerous.",由此归纳出,减肥不能一味节食,必须在节食和运动二者间找到平衡。

28. C 第三段第一句"A consistent pattern of daily physical activity and exercise is one of the healthiest habits you can get into."以及倒数第二句"And besides, exercise makes you feel wonderful, provided that you do not overdo it."表明,适量运动不仅是一种积极的生活方式,还可以给人带来愉悦的体验。段落中间则举例说明运动的各种形式。

29. D 第四段第一句"Vegetarianism is becoming increasingly popular among college students."为主题句,其余部分给出了数据说明,讨论选择素食的原因并提供了一些饮食建议,均为支撑细节。

30. E 第五段第一句"A healthy outlook about your body and appearance and how it relates to food and physical activity is very important for young adults."意指饮食和适量的运动对年轻人的健康非常重要,不要做有损健康的行为(Self-destructive behaviors),应尊重身体,善待身体(Keep your mind and body in shape by treating them both with respect)。

31. F 定位第一段第二句"It is reported that 8 of the 10 leading causes of death in America are directly related to what we eat and drink."。

32. D 定位第二段第四句"If you want to lose weight, the equation is simple, eat less and exercise more."。

33. A 定位第二段第七句"The easiest way to decrease the number of calories your body stores as fat is to not consume those calories in the first place; especially since it is much more difficult to burn calories once they are consumed."。

34. B 定位第四段第四句"Some people consider themselves vegetarian simply because they do not eat red meat."。

35. C 定位第五段最后一句"A healthy self-image and realistic perception of yourself is one of the healthiest feats you can achieve."。

Part Two

【文章大意】主要介绍慢性阻塞性肺病的症状、致病因素、发病机制、分类和改善途径。

【解题思路】

36. B 根据第五段第一、二句"COPD develops slowly. Symptoms often worsen over time and can limit your ability to do routine activities."选题。

37. D　第一段第二句"COPD can cause coughing that produces large amounts of mucus (a slimy substance), wheezing, shortness of breath, chest tightness, and other symptoms."指出慢性阻塞性肺病的症状包括咳痰、哮喘、气短和胸闷等,D选项提到的咳血则不是其症状。

38. A　文章第二段介绍了肺的工作原理,吸入的空气首先进入气管(windpipe),然后进入支气管(bronchial tubes),再进入由支气管分化成的细支气管(bronchioles),最后进入细支气管末端的肺泡(alveoli)。肺泡外面包绕着许多毛细血管,当吸入的空气到达肺泡时,空气中的氧气透过肺泡壁和毛细血管壁进入血液,同时血液中的二氧化碳也透过毛细血管壁和肺泡壁进入肺泡,随呼气的过程排出体外。

39. C　根据第四段第六、七、八句"In chronic bronchitis, the lining of the airways is constantly irritated and inflamed. This causes the lining to thicken. Lots of thick mucus forms in the airways, making it hard to breathe.",慢性支气管炎是由于支气管黏膜不断受到刺激而引发炎症,导致黏膜增厚及分泌物增多,引发呼吸困难。C项指出气道发炎因而变得狭窄或阻塞符合文章意思,其他三选项指出慢性阻塞性肺病发作时肺组织弹性增强、黏液减少以及与肺泡中无气体交换与原文第四段相悖。

40. C　第四段最后两句"Most people who have COPD have both emphysema and chronic bronchitis. Thus, the general term 'COPD' is more accurate."指出慢性阻塞性肺病患者同时患有肺气肿和慢性支气管炎,因此用"慢性阻塞性肺病"这一统称更为精确,而其他三个选项内容在文中均未给出。

41. C　参照文章第五段最后两句话"COPD has no cure yet, and doctors don't know how to reverse the damage to the airways and lungs. However, treatments and lifestyle changes can help you feel better, stay more active, and slow the progress of the disease.",慢性阻塞性肺病目前尚无治愈方法,但治疗和改变生活方式可以提高生活质量,减慢疾病进程。另外,本段还指出气道与肺泡的损害具有不可逆性,此病非传染性疾病等。因而A、B、D均为错误选项。

42. D　从第一段第三句"Cigarette smoking is the leading cause of COPD."得知A选项正确,根据第四段第一句"In the United States, the term 'COPD' includes two main conditions …"和第五段内容判断B、C选项正确,而D选项则为错误表述,因而是本题正确答案。

Part Three
【文章大意】文章报道了埃博拉病毒分型、感染途径与症状、病毒爆发史、致病致死性、治疗和疫苗研制情况,并从生物伦理角度阐述了埃博拉疫苗临床试验阶段有关使用人群的争议问题。

【解题思路】

43. C　题目意为国际卫生条例在西非告知于众,此信息在文中没有给出,故选C。

44. A　根据第二段第二句"The West Africa outbreak is from a new strain of the Zaire species, with a reported case-fatality rate of 55%.",题目正确。

45. B　根据第三段第二句"Human-to-human transmission occurs only by close contact with infected body fluids.",只有密切接触患者的体液才会在人与人之间传染,因此

题目错误。

46. B 根据第四段第五句"Of greatest concern is the potential urban spread, including capital cities.",城市疫情扩散存在潜在风险,但还没有发生疫情,所以题目错误。

47. A 根据第五段第二句"There are no licensed vaccines or specific antivirals or immune-mediated treatments for ill patients or for postexposure prophylaxis.",题目正确。

48. B 第六段最后一句"... is the ethical concern of administering an experimental drug to African patients that has not undergone any safety testing in humans."和第七段第六句"Liberian officials apparently did not approve the use of an investigational drug administered in their territory.",对非洲患者使用试验性病毒抗体既存在伦理上的问题,又存在事实上的阻力,所以题目是错误的。

49. C 第六段第一句"... 2 US aid workers infected in Liberia were treated with an experimental anti-Ebola antibody prior to being transported to Atlanta.",2 名美国救援人员被运送到亚特兰大前注射了测试性埃博拉病毒抗体,并未提及治疗后痊愈。故选 C。

50. A 文章第七段从生物伦理角度谈论疫苗在试验阶段进行治疗的种种问题,根据首尾两句话得知题目是正确的。

Part Four

【文章大意】文章阐述了过量服用阿司匹林中毒的种类,成人和儿童服用阿司匹林注意事项,过量服用阿司匹林而导致急慢性中毒的症状、处理方法以及避免过量服用或误食阿司匹林的建议。

【解题思路】

51. A 第一段第一句为段落主题句,指出过量服用阿司匹林中毒有两种类型。第二句是关于急性阿司匹林中毒的内容。第三、四句是关于过量服用阿司匹林慢性中毒及原因的内容。A 选项是关于阿司匹林慢性中毒易发人群的内容,为合理选项。有助于正确选题的重要词句包括:there are two forms of which/In acute aspirin poisoning/Another form of aspirin overdose is called chronic overdose/The chronic form。

52. D 第二段第二句"In children, aspirin is not recommended, though some kids with heart conditions may be on very low dose amounts to prevent blood clotting."谈到不推荐儿童服用阿司匹林,一些患有心脏疾病的儿童服用阿司匹林抗血凝时应注意低剂量使用。D 选项接着指出具体的低剂量值。重要词汇为 low dose amounts/Low-dose aspirin。

53. C 第四段谈到人们处理阿司匹林中毒的具体方法和注意事项。作为本段第一句,C 选项指出"急、慢性阿司匹林中毒都是紧急医疗事件,需要即刻进行医疗救助",是下面三句话内容的主旨概括,是本段的主题句。重要词汇:need immediate attention/should/should not/and it is not advisable to/should。

54. B 第五段谈及人们在配合医疗人员救治中毒者时可以提供患者的一些信息,B 选项在首句作为概括全段的主题句最为合理。内容和信息相关。重要词句:they can help greatly by having some information/If they know/this is great information/but whatever extra information can be given may prove helpful。

55. E 第七段第二句"Many companies still make forms of baby aspirin that are chewable."指出很多公司目前还生产婴儿服用的阿司匹林咀嚼片;E 选项接着讲述儿童喜

欢这种阿司匹林的口味,因而也就容易过量服用;下一句"If there are adults(or kids with heart defects) that use the chewable form,keep these medications far out of reach of other children."说要把阿司匹林咀嚼片放在儿童接触不到的地方。内容都和儿童相关。重要词汇:"baby"aspirin/kids/children。

Part Five

【文章大意】文章介绍了运用激光手术治疗近视的原理、手术过程及术后注意事项。

【解题思路】

56. A contact lenses:隐形眼镜,其他几个选项表达不准确。

57. C vision:视觉、视力。20/20 vision,也可写为 twenty-twenty/20—20 vision:非常好的视力(the ability to see perfectly)。第一段主要内容是关于激光手术如何矫正视力,最后一句话的意思是:许多患者接受激光治疗后视力变得非常好。

58. B attach 与 to 固定搭配,意为"与……连接在一起"。The laser system includes a large machine with a microscope attached to it and a computer screen. 表示"此激光设备包括一台连接着显微镜和电脑视频的大型仪器"。clip:夹住;fasten 扣住,捆住;implement:实施,执行。

59. C 根据"you may feel the pressure and experience some discomfort during this part of the procedure",说明此时视力应该是"变模糊",才会让人有压迫(pressure)和不适感(discomfort),故选 C。blur:变模糊;flag:衰退。

60. C Laser energy is focused inside the cornea tissue,which creates thousands of small bubbles of gas and water that expand and connect to separate the tissue underneath the cornea surface,creating a flap. 此句句意为:"激光脉冲聚集到角膜组织中,产生成千上万的水泡和气泡并不断扩展,分离角膜组织,形成相应的分离面。"在"组织里面"产生水泡和气泡,然后"膨胀扩大(expand)",故选 C。

61. D You will be able to see,but you will experience fluctuating degrees of blurred vision during the rest of the procedure. 此句句意为:"术中你可以看见东西,但会出现不同程度的视力模糊,有时严重,有时程度稍轻。"选 D:"波动性的",符合句意。additive:成瘾的;agonizing:使人痛苦的;flexible:灵活的。

62. A 此处译为:"一旦激光准备好,这种光可以使眼球固定在一个位置。"选 A 符合语句逻辑。

63. D As the laser removes corneal tissue,some people have reported a smell similar to burning hair. 此句意思:"当激光刀移除角膜组织时,有人说有像头发烧焦了的气味。"选 D 句意合理。screen:筛查;scrape:刮,擦;implant:植入;remove:移除,摘除。

64. D Before the start of surgery,your doctor will have programmed the computer to vaporize a particular amount of tissue based on the measurements taken at your initial evaluation. 此处译为:"根据术前的测量设定电脑程序,术中蒸发一定数量的角膜组织。"assessments、evaluations 和 estimations:对形势、情况、状况等做出的判断、评估、评价等;measurements:测量、测定;take measurements 为固定搭配。

65. C ... protect your eye from accidentally being hit or poked ... 此句译为:"防止眼睛受到意外碰撞或戳刺。"其他选项均不符合常理或逻辑。

11

III　Writing

66.【范文】

Recent years have seen great progress in China's medical reform, but people still find it difficult and expensive to see a doctor.

This phenomenon can be attributed to the following three factors, among others. The first one is the uneven distribution of medical care resources. People often take a lot of time and trouble in getting treatment in good but overcrowded hospitals in big cities. Second, current medical insurance and pricing systems still have defects. Unreasonable medicines and check-up fees increase most patients' financial burden, and those with serious illnesses are often reduced to poverty. To make matters worse, such hospital malpractices as bad service attitude, giving excessive medical treatment and receiving patients' red envelopes increase the mental and economic pressures for patients, making their experience of seeing a doctor a painful nightmare.

China must deepen its medical care reform by optimizing the distribution of medical resources, changing the medicines pricing mechanism and improving medical workers' professional ethics, letting every Chinese citizen enjoy the benefit of convenient and cheap health care service. (172 words)

【审题】

写作部分要求根据给定的情景——中国目前存在"看病难看病贵"的现象进行写作，要求分析造成这种现象的原因、列举解决问题的对策。文章应属说明文，除遵守说明文写作的基本要求外，写作中的一个重点和难点是如何正确写出一些涉及医疗卫生领域话题的英语表达，如"医疗改革、医疗卫生资源、看病、医疗保险、药费、大病、服务态度、过度治疗、收红包、医疗卫生服务、医疗卫生职业道德"等。

【范文评析】

文章首先根据作文任务给定的信息，直奔主题，指出目前存在的一种社会现象，以问题的提出开头。文章的重点放在问题成因的剖析上：第二段第一句总领全段，随后从三个方面给出具体的原因。第三段简明扼要，列举了解决问题的三个办法。

文章结构层次清晰，主题表达明确，阐述部分充分合理，每个主题句都有适当的扩展或说明；熟练使用 first, second 和 To make matters worse 等词语衔接手段，正确运用医学话题相关的一些词汇表达；现在分词短语状语结构的使用(making their experience of seeing a doctor a painful nightmare/letting every Chinese citizen enjoy the benefit of convenient and cheap health care service)则是本文句子中的一个亮点。

医护英语水平考试(三级)
模拟训练(二)

听力文本

This is METS-3 listening test. There are four parts in the test. You will hear each part twice. We will now stop for a moment before we start the test. Please ask any questions now because you must not speak during the test. Now, look at the instructions for Part One.

You will hear five extracts from conversations taking place in different clinical departments. Choose which case each doctor is discussing from the list A—F. Use each letter A—F only once. There is one extra letter which you do not need to use. Mark the corresponding letter on your answer sheet. You will hear each extract twice. Now we are ready to start.

Extract 1

You will need to take some medication home with you. I have prescribed some tablets for your blood pressure and you need to take one twice a day morning and evening. I have also prescribed a sublingual tablet which you should take when the pain comes in your chest. Just put one tablet under your tongue and let it dissolve. You must only take a maximum of two tablets a day.

Extract 2

The ankle is very swollen and it is possible that there may be some bleeding within the joint. You need to have a support bandage applied by the nurse. You must keep the foot elevated as much as you can for 3 days or until the swelling goes down and your ankle feels better. You should have a week off. If your ankle isn't better in a week, please come back to see me.

Extract 3

Now we're moving on to examine your arms and legs neurologically. Start by putting both arms out in the air in front of you and shut your eyes. Hold the arms still while I look at them. Now wiggle your fingers as though you were playing the piano. Open your eyes, and make a pointer by stretching out your index finger. Now touch my finger and then touch your nose. Now try this on the other side.

Extract 4

Well, we were told that his lungs were immature because he was preterm, and he needed to have help with his breathing with a machine. I do know, Doctor, though, that he had extra problems because he had an infection and he also became jaundiced, and at the time the doctor explained to me that they thought he may have developed jaundice both because he was premature and also because he had some bleeding in the brain.

Extract 5

Could you please get into a gown and I'll examine you ... I think that there is a good possibility that you have appendicitis although we cannot be sure. We'll get some blood tests looking at your white blood count. However, based on your symptoms I think it would be wise to admit you to hospital, and start you on an IV, and if you don't improve, then I think we should remove the appendix.

Now you'll hear Part One again. This is the end of Part One. Now look at Part Two. You will hear a conversation between the student nurse Barbara and her instructor, Mrs. Baker. For each of the following statements, decide whether it is True or False. If there is not enough information to answer True or False, choose Not Given. Mark the corresponding letter on your answer sheet. You will hear the recording twice.

Barbara: Mrs. Baker, I will be taking care of the patient in Room 322 Bed 2. Here is the care plan.

Mrs. Baker: All right. When did the patient have the surgery?

Barbara: He was sent to the OR early in the morning and had a cholecystectomy. He came back to the floor at about 12 o'clock.

Mrs. Baker: He is a fresh post-operative patient. It's a very good case for you to learn post-operative care.

Barbara: Yes.

Mrs. Baker: What kind of procedure did he have?

Barbara: Cholecystectomy.

Mrs. Baker: I know, but was it open or laparoscopic?

Barbara: Oh, sorry. He had an open cholecystectomy.

Mrs. Baker: You should indicate the procedure in your care plan because the care would not be the same when the procedure is different.

Barbara: Yes. Thank you.

Mrs. Baker: Tell me what your focus of care would be.

Barbara: Pain, incision care, vital signs, circulation and perfusion ...

Mrs. Baker: A little bit more detailed?

Barbara:	Like all post-operative patients, the patient will be in pain. Right now he has patient controlled analgesia (PCA) running morphine. The PCA is expected to be replaced by PRN IV push or PO pills by tomorrow morning.
Mrs. Baker:	Good.
Barbara:	I will check vital signs every 30 minutes for two hours, then every one hour for four hours, then every four hours two times. This is the routine for all post-operative patient care.
Mrs. Baker:	OK. If the vitals are not within the normal limits, what do you do?
Barbara:	Recheck the patient first. If it is confirmed the vital signs are not within the normal limits, I will call the doctor. For example, if the temperature is above 100 degrees, I will call.
Mrs. Baker:	All right, you also need to initiate some nursing care to help the patient.
Barbara:	Right, such as checking the incision, monitoring the labs, giving PRN meds, putting an ice pack ...
Mrs. Baker:	Another very important post-operative nursing care activity is to help the patient cough effectively.
Barbara:	Yes. I forgot to put that in my care plan. I will do patient teaching on how to use the incentive spirometer.
Mrs. Baker:	Why do we encourage coughing after surgery?
Barbara:	To reduce the chance of getting pneumonia, which is one of the most common complications of surgery.
Mrs. Baker:	Right, coughing will help expand the lungs and clear the airway. It's an evidence-based practice that significantly reduces post-operative pneumonia.
Barbara:	Yes, I should have put it in the plan. I'll fix the care plan and turn it in to you a little bit later. Is that all right?
Mrs. Baker:	All right.

Now you'll hear Part Two again. This is the end of Part Two. Now look at Part Three. You will hear a ward team meeting among four nurses discussing a patient with stroke. For questions 14—20, choose the most appropriate answer. Mark the corresponding letter on your answer sheet. You will hear the discussion twice.

Andrea: Let's start with Lidia. Lidia's an 80-year-old Russian lady who's been living in her own home for 40 years; she's a very independent woman. You might remember that her daughters had visited her on a Sunday morning as usual and found her to be uncoordinated; um, she was having trouble picking up her cup of tea. They noticed that she was slurring her speech as well. Lidia said she'd had a "funny turn" the night before, unfortunately, by the time they brought her to hospital it was well over the initial three hours from the onset of the stroke.

15

She's been with us for two weeks now and has been working really hard with everyone so that she can get back to her own home. The purpose of this meeting is for us to report back on what we've all been doing for Lidia. Then we need to finalize her discharge plan. William, do you want to kick off?

William: Mm, I examined her yesterday, and I feel that she's doing well medically. I asked her about her goals and going home seems to be top of the list.

Andrea: Yes, she's spoken to me about how she was managing at home before the stroke. At this moment, she'll need a lot of help with her ADLs (activities of daily living). Kim, how did you find her?

Kim: I agree with both of you. She's been trying really hard. She's been doing all the physio exercises I give her. I'm a little concerned about her ability to perform the basic ADLs, especially showering, toileting, eating and mobility.

William: Yes, I'm a bit worried about that as well. Um, why don't we have a look at the home assessment? Has the Occupational Therapist team done a home assessment yet?

Andrea: Not yet. I've booked a home assessment with Occupational Therapy on Monday, 12th June. That'll give us a better idea about the sort of modifications which need to be made for safety and to allow her to be as independent as possible.

Kim: Good. I'm pleased with her progress. The weakness on her left side has partially resolved. Unfortunately, she's still got a bit of trouble with vision loss on that side. I've been training her to turn to the left to look for anything she might run into.

Andrea: Um, Lidia's going to stay with her daughter until the safety modifications in the house are finished.

William: That's good. Tina, what about speech and language therapy? How's she doing?

Tina: Well, my role has been to help Lidia's swallow reflex. I've been concentrating on her swallowing problem and speech difficulties. Remember she had quite a lot of difficulty swallowing when she first came in.

Andrea: Yes, her nutritional status was quite poor. She wasn't used to the food they serve in hospital.

Tina: No, it's very different from her usual diet. Her daughters brought in the food she likes. She still has some tongue and lip weakness. It's quite hard for her to speak properly. I've been practicing a lot of mouth exercises with her, and she's certainly improving. She's always been a very social person, so the ability to communicate is important to her.

William: Have you referred her for speech and language therapy after discharge?

Tina: No, I haven't referred her to a Speech Therapist yet. That's part of the referral to the District Nurses. Andrea, you've organized that, haven't you?

Andrea: Not yet. I wanted to wait until the team meeting is finished. I'll ring this afternoon. So, can we put Lidia's expected date of discharge down as Friday, 9 June?

Now you'll hear Part Three again. This is the end of Part Three. Now look at Part Four. You will hear a speech on the prostate removal. Complete the notes below by filling each space 21—25 with a single word. Write the answers on your answer sheet. You will hear the speech twice.

Male: In older men it is quite common for the prostate to enlarge and cause the symptoms you've been experiencing. To relieve these symptoms, it may be necessary to remove the prostate but there are some drugs which may help. Unfortunately, I don't think the drugs will help in your case so we'll have to operate.

Before your operation, I would like to explain what happens when your prostate gland is removed. You'll have a few tests before your operation, like blood and urine tests, heart tracing, a chest X-ray and sometimes an IVP, intravenous pyelogram, which means we'll inject some contrasting dye into your vein which will pass through the kidneys and then we'll take some X-rays of your kidneys. You will speak to an anesthetist who will decide on your type of anesthesia—a general when you would be completely asleep or an epidural which only numbs the lower part of your body.

There are two ways of removing the prostate. One is by operating after inserting a telescope through the penis or by making a cut in the lower abdomen. I'll decide which method to use after I've examined you.

After the operation your urine would be drained by a tube called an indwelling catheter. You may have some blood in the tube. Your bladder would be washed with water. You'll also have a tube in your arm called IV which may supply you with saline or blood.

It's recommended that you start drinking large quantities of fluid after the operation. You can have tea, coffee, squash or water but fizzy drinks are not recommended. This will speed up your recovery and wash away the blood in the catheter.

The bladder tube will be removed two to five days after the operation. You should continue to drink as much as possible and pass water every two or three hours. Depending on your recovery, you are usually allowed home after about five days. Drink a lot of liquids at home and we'll give you stool softener to avoid constipation. If you have any problems, call your doctor.

Your sex life will change a little. You can have intercourse a few weeks after the operation, but you will not emit any semen from your penis at sexual climax. Your semen will flow into your bladder and your urine may be cloudy after intercourse.

You are unlikely to produce any further children but should not rely on this as safe contraception.

Now you'll hear Part Four again. This is the end of Part Four. You now have five minutes to write your answers on the answer sheet. You have one more minute. This is the end of the test.

参考答案与试题评析

I Listening

Part One

1.【语段大意】医生正对患者进行指导用药：针对血压的片剂，一日早晚两次，一次一片；针对胸部疼痛发作时的片剂，舌下给药(sublingual tablet)，一日最多(a maximum of)两片。

【解题思路】D 可听到 medication, blood pressure, pain comes in your chest 等关键信息。

2.【语段大意】患者踝部(ankle)水肿(swollen)，可能关节内有积血，医生建议使用绷带支撑(support bandage)，足部抬高进行消肿，如不见缓解，须再次就医。

【解题思路】C 可听到 ankle is very swollen, support bandage 等关键信息。

3.【语段大意】医生通过指导患者闭眼举臂，挥动手臂或指物等动作对患者进行双臂双腿神经检查(examine your arms and legs neurologically)。

【解题思路】A 可听到 examine, arms and legs, neurologically 等关键信息。

4.【语段大意】患者为一早产(preterm)发育不全(immature)婴儿，须呼吸机辅助呼吸，且出现感染(infection)与黄疸(jaundice)，怀疑黄疸原因为早产及脑部出血(some bleeding in the brain)。

【解题思路】F 可听到 immature, preterm, infection, jaundiced 等关键信息。

5.【语段大意】本题描述的是医生检查完患者后，发现患者极可能患有阑尾炎(appendicitis)，建议其住院接受静脉药物治疗(on an Ⅳ)，如无效，则将采取手术。

【解题思路】B 可听到 appendicitis, admit you to hospital, remove the appendix 等关键信息。

Part Two

【语篇大意】护理实习生跟指导护士之间的对话。

【解题思路】

6. A 护理实习生 Barbara 负责 322 房间 2 床病人的护理，信息正确，故答案为 A。

7. B 病人所做的是开腹胆囊切除术(open cholecystectomy)，不是胃部手术，故答案选 B。

8. B 该病人做的是开腹胆囊切除术(open cholecystectomy)，不是腹腔镜胆囊切除术(laparoscopic cholecystectomy)，故答案选 B。

9. A 开腹胆囊切除术和腹腔镜胆囊切除术的术后护理是不相同的,故答案选 A。

10. C 腹腔镜胆囊切除术作为胆结石(gallstones)病人的首选疗法已经取代了开腹胆囊切除术,句子本身并没有错,但对话中并没有提及,故答案选 C。

11. A 术后病人的护理重点包括疼痛护理、切口护理、监测生命体征、循环和灌注,描述与对话中完全一致,故答案选 A。

12. A 帮助术后病人有效咳嗽非常重要,因为有效咳嗽能减少术后肺炎的发病率,题目中描述完全正确,故答案选 A。

13. B 咳嗽有益于肺部扩张(expand)、清洁气道,不是收缩肺部,故答案选 B。

Part Three

【语篇大意】病人 Lidia 因中风住院一段时间后即将出院,康复病房的四位护士就 Lidia 的治疗进展召开的一次会议。

【解题思路】

14. C 本题是关于病人 Lidia 的基本情况,她是一位 80 岁的独居老人,俄罗斯人,显然答案为 C。

15. B 本题是问 Lidia 的主要疾病,讨论中多次提到 Lidia 是因为中风住院的,所以答案为 B。

16. A 本题是问 Lidia 什么时候被送到医院的,在病历介绍中提到她是在一个周日上午被女儿发现的,送到医院时已经过了中风发作的最初三小时,据此可推断她是在中风发作后的几小时被送到医院的,答案为 A。

17. B 本题是针对讨论中这句话 "I asked her about her goals and going home seems to be top of the list" 而命题的,显然 Lidia 是想回到自己的家中,答案为 B。

18. C 本题问家庭评估(home assessment)预约的时间,Andrea 明确提到是 6 月 12 日,周一,答案 B 中的 6 月 9 日,周五,是预计出院日期,故本题答案为 C。

19. A 本题是关于 Lidia 出院后住处的问题,讨论中明确提到她将和女儿住在一起直到房屋安全改进完成。本题答案为 A。

20. B 本题三个选项中,A 是关于 Lidia 的视力问题,她的左眼视力受到影响,不是右眼,选项 A 错误。选项 C 中 Tina has already referred Lidia to a Speech Therapist 与文中不符,故本题答案为 B。

Part Four

【语篇大意】关于前列腺切除手术的介绍。

【解题思路】

21. enlarge 此处为介绍开头提到老年人常见前列腺(the prostate)肥大(enlarge),并引起一系列症状。所以此处应填 enlarge。

22. intravenous 文中讲述到医生认为针对此患者的前列腺肥大,药物治疗无效,建议考虑手术。在手术前,先做一系列检查,包括血液检查、尿液检查、心脏检查(heart tracing)、胸部 X 光以及静脉内肾盂造影(intravenous pyelogram)。所以此处应填 intravenous。

23. anesthesia 文中讲述到手术前须与麻醉师(anesthetist)讨论麻醉类型(type of anesthesia),一类是全身(general)麻醉,患者手术时处于安睡状态;一类是硬膜外(epidural)麻醉,仅麻醉下半身。根据短文内容,此处应填 anesthesia。

24. telescope　文中讲述到两种切除前列腺的方法,一种从阴茎处(penis)插入手术操作镜(telescope),一种在下腹部(the lower abdomen)直接开口。故此处应填 telescope。

25. indwelling　文中提到在术后,尿液通过导尿管排泄,导尿管因插至下体内,并留置,所以称为 indwelling catheter。故此处应填 indwelling。

Ⅱ　Reading

Part One

【文章大意】文章介绍了几种关于人们为何打呵欠的不同解释,以及打呵欠为何具有传染性的研究结果。

【解题思路】

26. B　第一段段首"We do know lots of interesting things about yawning"介绍了关于打呵欠有很多有趣的说法,段中与段尾"scientists are discovering there's more to yawning than most people think","However, there are several theories about why we yawn."指出关于为何打呵欠还有更多的科学发现。

27. A　第二段段首"Scientists propose that our bodies induce yawning to draw in more oxygen or remove a buildup of carbon dioxide."介绍有科学家指出打呵欠是人体排出二氧化碳,获得更多氧气的一种途径,可见这是从生理的角度探讨打呵欠的原因。

28. F　第三段首句"Some think that yawning began with our ancestors, who used yawning to show their teeth and intimidate others."介绍了一种观点,即祖先们打呵欠是为了以露齿的行为威吓对手,以及下文衍生出的理论"An offshoot of this theory is the idea that yawning developed from early man as a signal for us to change activities."早期人类打呵欠很可能是作为一种提示的信号。由此得知,此段是从进化论的角度来谈论打呵欠的原因。

29. D　第四段段首"A more recent theory proposed ... it's a way to cool down their brains.",以及段中"In 2007, researchers ... proposed that yawning may be a means to keep the brain cool."介绍了有研究认为,打呵欠是为了冷却大脑。故依据这一提法作答。

30. C　第五段首句"Recent studies show contagious yawning may be linked to one's capacity for empathy."介绍了打呵欠有传染性可能与人的共情力有关,并在下文以对自闭症儿童和正常儿童的呵欠实验证明了这一观点。故据此选择。

31. F　定位第一段第一句话"We do know lots of interesting things about yawning: you start yawning in uterus ... ",uterus 意思是"子宫",即是指出生前就开始打呵欠,故选 F。

32. A　定位第二段第三句话"Larger groups produce more carbon dioxide, which means our bodies would act to draw in more oxygen and get rid of the excess carbon dioxide.",处理掉过量的二氧化碳与"exhale excessive carbon dioxide"呼出多余的二氧化碳之意相符,故选 A。

33. D　定位第三段最后一句话"Therefore, the 'contagious' yawn could be an instinctual reaction to a signal from one member of the 'herd' reminding the others to stay alert.",是本能的反应,故选 D。

34. C 定位第四段第二句话"In 2007，researchers，including a professor of psychology，from the University of Albany proposed that yawning may be a means to keep the brain cool."，打呵欠是给大脑降温，保持大脑"凉爽"的一种途径，对应选项 C，"regulation of brain temperature"，调节大脑温度。

35. E 定位第五段第五句话"Since autism is a disorder that affects a person's social interaction skills，including the ability to empathize with others，the autistic kids' lack of yawning when watching others do so could indicate they're less empathetic."，自闭儿童共情力差，故而少有受群体或环境感染而打呵欠的行为。对应选项 E。

Part Two

【文章大意】本文在介绍阻塞性睡眠呼吸暂停综合征的影响因素和症状的基础上，指出不同类型的阻塞性睡眠呼吸暂停综合征诱因不同，不同人群患病风险不同。同时介绍了通过多导睡眠图技术研究睡眠呼吸暂停综合征，并提出了行为治疗、CPAP 设备治疗和内置 UAS 等治疗方法。

【解题思路】

36. B 第一段第五句话"With sleep apnea，your breathing pauses multiple times during sleep."指出 sleep apnea 意为"呼吸暂停"，故对应选项"without breath"。

37. D 第一段第六句话"The pauses can last from a few seconds to minutes and can occur more than five times per hour，to as high as 100 times per hour（Fewer than five times per hour is normal.）"括号中明确指出，每小时少于五次属于正常，故选项 D"每小时四次"正确。

38. C 第二段第一句话"Obstructive sleep apnea，the most common type，is caused by a blockage of the airway，usually when the soft tissue in the back of the throat collapses."指出气道阻塞是诱因，而这种情况常常出现于咽后部的软组织塌陷。据此作答。

39. B 第三段前两句话"Sleep apnea is almost twice as common in men as it is in women. Other risk factors include：being overweight，being over age 40，smoking and so on."介绍了男性较女性更易出现睡眠呼吸暂停，另外，超重、吸烟、年龄超过 40 等也是危险因素，因而选 B。

40. A 第五段首句"The first line of defense can be behavioral."介绍了以改变行为方式治疗睡眠呼吸暂停综合征，相关行为包括"weight loss""stop using alcohol or medicines"，即减重、戒酒与停止服用令人嗜睡的药物等。四个选项中只有 A 未提及。

41. D 第七段最后一句话"The Inspire device is surgically implanted below the collarbone and works with ..."指出这种呼吸装置是通过外科手术植入锁骨下方，因而是创伤性的手术；根据第六段最后两句话"CPAP use mild air pressure to keep your airways open. The air is delivered through a mask that fits over your nose and mouth，or only your nose."得知 CPAP 和 UAS 毫无相似点，因而 B 选项表述错误，而 A、C 两项均未提及。据此，只有 D 为正确的推论。

42. C 根据第二段"Obstructive sleep apnea，the most common type，is caused by ... The less common form，central sleep apnea，happens if ..."判断 A 选项错误；根据第三段第一句话"Sleep apnea is almost twice as common in men as it is in women."判断 B 选项错

误;第九段讨论的是 UAS 治疗睡眠呼吸暂停的原理和使用方法,因而该段最后一句话"The patient turns the system on before going to sleep and off upon waking, using a remote control."中"the system"指的是"UAS",故 D 错误;第七段第三句话"The Inspire Upper Airway System (UAS) is intended for consumers with moderate to severe OSA …"指出适合 UAS 手术的病患群体,因而 C 选项正确。

Part Three

【文章大意】这是一份病理检验专业的推介说明,介绍了课程目标、教学师生比、课程学制、学习内容、教学方法、实习和就业前景等。

【解题思路】

43. A 在"Year two"关于第二学年学习内容与目标的介绍中指出"All of these tests aid in the diagnosis of all types of diseases.",据此,病理检验所涉及的各种检验对诊断各类疾病均有辅助功能。题干说法正确。

44. C 在"Career outlook"中指出"There is a high demand for technicians to work in … and large private pathology providers …"没有提到 medical universities 有大量技术人员需求。故而题干说法错误。

45. B "Working with industry"标题下第一段第一句话"You will undertake 20 days of work experience during the second year, organized by RMIT."指出,第二学年里的实习时间仅为 20 天,而非整学年。题干说法错误。

46. A "City campus"标题下第四段第一句话"Class sizes are small and the staff-to-student ratio in laboratories allows opportunities for individual teaching."指出小班教学与实验室师生比为个体化教学提供了保障。题干说法正确。

47. C "Pathways"标题下"Graduates of the Diploma of Laboratory Technology (Pathology Testing) who are successful in gaining a place are eligible to apply for exemptions of up to one year (96 credit points) from the following programs."指出,病检毕业生成功考取以下专业有资格申请免修 96 学时的课程,而题干意为学生要完成所有课程方可申请期末考试免考,文中没有涉及此信息。题干说法错误。

48. B "Year one"标题下第一段"The first year provides you with a foundation …"和"Year two"标题下第一段"The second year involves more specialized study …"分别指出,学生在第一学年主要学习基础课程,而在第二学年才会学习更多的专业课程。题干说法错误。

49. A "Year two"标题下第二段第一句话"You will learn the skills to …, as well as how to prepare thin slices of liver and other tissues to examine microscopically."指出,学生在第二学年中习得如何准备肝脏薄片和其他组织切片用于显微镜检查,故毕业生具备该能力。题干说法正确。

50. C "Professional recognition"一段中首句"Students are eligible for student membership of the Australian Society for Microbiology and …"指出,学生有资格申请加入澳大利亚微生物学协会。题干说法,所有学生都一定是病理学协会成员,文中未提及。

Part Four

【文章大意】文章介绍了有关安慰剂的争议、安慰剂的效应原理、经典条件反射和预期效应对安慰剂效应的作用,并罗列了安慰剂被当作万能药剂的诸多事例。

【解题思路】

51. E 文章开篇指出,Moerman 和 Jonas 认为将安慰剂效应定义为一种生理效应不合逻辑,因为安慰剂成分并无任何直接效用,并在下文进一步提出使用安慰剂是不道德的。E 选项表达了 Moerman 和 Jonas 的看法,衔接紧密、逻辑合理。

52. B 此段段首介绍了 Irving Kirsch 的猜想,即安慰剂效应来源于预期效应中的自我满足效应。结合所缺部分之后的两句,它们分别讨论了经典条件反射和预期效应对安慰剂效应的作用,因此缺失部分应为关于经典条件反射和预期效应的承接句,"Both conditioning and expectations play a role in placebo effect"为合理衔接,因而选 B。

53. C 所缺部分的上句提到,研究发现,患者对安慰剂应答率的提高来自医生的关怀、关注和信心;所缺部分的下句又再次提及患者的信念也会对安慰剂效应有影响。作为承接句,应选择预期效应的发生与一系列因素有关,因而选 C。

54. A 此段首句指出,如果患者被告知他们的预期不现实或者安慰剂无效,安慰剂就不会起作用,这是因为安慰剂效应是建立在预期和条件反射基础上的。A 选项"一旦向患者解释了这种效应机制,条件反射式的疼痛缓和效果就会完全消失"则是对以上理论的举例说明,因而是合理衔接。

55. F 此段首句为主题句,指出安慰剂的万能,被当作肌肉松弛剂、兴奋剂、镇静剂等,并给出了例子,如所缺部分的上句以"安慰剂可以帮助吸烟者戒烟"举例说明安慰剂效应,下一句可能仍是举例,F 选项则是举例说明想象中的过敏原导致过敏的情况,与前面例子呈并列关系,是合理衔接。

Part Five

【文章大意】文章介绍了基因能够决定人对药物的反应,科学家通过药物基因组学研究发现基因变异与药物毒理之间的联系。由此指出,未来对药物基因组学的研究能够有助于医生为患者开出更为有效的药物,尽可能避免药物的毒副作用。

【解题思路】

56. D 基因决定高矮、发色,基因同样能够决定人对药物的反应,D 项正确。predict:预测;diagnose:诊断;calculate:计算,均不合适。

57. C 上文介绍了基因决定人对药物的反应,随着药物进入体内,药物和蛋白质相互作用,C 项正确。contact:联系,connect:连接,均不合理;act:行动,不与 with 连接。

58. A 科学家希望能够帮助医生视不同的个体来开处方。prescribe:开药方;deliberate:慎重的,仔细考虑;describe:描绘;banner:旗帜,标语。

59. A 上句说明一些药物给部分病人带来严重的副作用,这句话则举例副作用,可描述副作用的只有 A 选项,toxic:有毒的。"可待因作为止疼药对 10% 的病人无效以及一种抗癌药物对极少部分人毒性甚强。"其他选项为 effective:有效果的;beneficial:有利的;fierce:猛烈的。

60. B "这一认知使得研究者迅速定位酶的基因变体,正是这种变体导致了危险反应的发生。"依据句意,只有介词 as 符合逻辑和搭配。

61. D "一些制药公司采集了临床病人的 DNA",这样的行为应该是在得到受试者同意之后,故依据句意,只能选 After。

62. B "药物基因组学研究者们已经识别出了很多基因因变异而影响了药物应答。"下一句"others"代指上句中的"genes",意指"药物基因组学研究者们也知道何处可以找到更多的此类基因",且"others"后连接了一个定语从句,关系代词 that 在从句中做宾语被省略。从句中,"be bound to"为固定短语,表示"必然",从句意为"那些基因是研究者们未来必然会发现的"。

63. C 此部分为非限制性定语从句,以 which 指代"人类基因组序列",从句部分在全句中不充当成分,只用来补充信息。

64. C "未来药物基因组学将使得医生初次诊疗就能给病人开出正确的药及正确的剂量。"为此句动词"使得"加上一个合适的副词,只有 increasingly 表示能力渐增。其他选项意思为 seriously:严重地、认真地;therapeutically:治疗上地;exclusively:专有地。

65. A 此处指识别药物毒副作用的基因基础将会使得常见救命药继续使用下去。常见救命药为 frequently lifesaving medications,其余选项意思为 consequently:因此;infrequently:罕见地;undoubtedly:毋庸置疑地。

Ⅲ Writing

66.【范文】

Should Nurses Go Abroad to Work?

Many Chinese nurses want to go abroad to work. According to the result of an online questionnaire, 81% of the respondents, most of whom are university nursing students, say that they want to work in a hospital in the USA or Australia.

There are at least two reasons behind this phenomenon. First of all, nurses in some developed countries are very highly paid. It is said that in Australia, for example, a nurse with a working experience of 5 or 6 years can earn as much as 60,000 Australian dollars a year. Secondly, working in a foreign country gives nurses much needed experience. This will certainly add some weight to their resumes and help them find better job opportunities when they return to China.

Considering the benefits working overseas might bring, Chinese nurses' enthusiasm to work abroad should not be dampened. But nursing abroad can also pose a number of challenges like the culture difference and the language barrier. Nurses need to think twice before they make the final decision. (177 words)

【审题】

写作部分要求根据给定的话题"中国很多护士选择出国工作的现象"进行写作。本部分给出段落提示句,要求先提出这一现象,然后分析造成这种现象的原因,最后阐明自己关于这一现象的看法。文章的主体部分在第二、三两段,要求考生对这一社会现象进行解释并加以评论,第二部分一般使用列举法,要注意第三部分段落扩展的三种常见方法:同意的观点、反对的观点、折中的观点。

【范文评析】

文章根据段落提示句,第一段首句开门见山,指出目前存在的一种社会现象,而后列举统计数据加以支撑。文章的重点放在第二段的原因分析及第三段的作者观点阐述上。第二段第一句总领全段,随后从两个方面给出具体的原因,使用了举例子、列数据的方式,增强说服力。第三段简明扼要,从正反两方面表达观点,以 but 作为转折,既看到了护士出国就业的优势及热情,也不能忽视其中的困难和挑战。

文章主题明确,结构清晰,层次分明,阐述部分客观全面,每个主题句都有适当的扩展或说明;正确使用 first of all, secondly 等列举用语,准确运用国外就业话题相关的一些词汇表达;句式多样,灵活运用了非限制性定语从句(most of whom are university nursing students)、插入语(for example)、现在分词状语结构(Considering the benefits working overseas might bring);词汇短语水平上的亮点有:as much as, add some weight to, pose a number of challenges, think twice before 等。

医护英语水平考试(三级)
模拟训练(三)

听力文本

This is METS-3 listening test. There are four parts in the test. Part One, Two, Three, and Four. You will hear each part twice. We will now stop for a moment before we start the test. Please ask any questions now because you must not speak during the test. Now, look at the instructions for Part One.

You will hear five extracts from conversations taking place in different clinical departments. Choose which case each doctor is discussing from the list A—F. Use each letter A—F only once. There is one extra letter which you do not need to use. Mark the corresponding letter on your answer sheet. You will hear each extract twice. Now we are ready to start.

Extract 1

A 55-year-old housewife, who had been well until four months ago, complained of tiredness and malaise. She had gained 9 kg in weight in the year before she presented to her GP although she denied eating more than usual. She was constipated and she noticed that her hair had started to fall out.

Extract 2

A 48-year-old man is noted to have a 2-day history of sore throat, subjective fever at home, and no medical illnesses. He denies cough or nausea. On examination, his temperature is 38.3 °C, and he has some tonsillar swelling but no exudates. He has bilateral enlarged and tender lymph nodes of the neck. The rapid streptococcal antigen test is negative.

Extract 3

A 22-year-old student was admitted to hospital with a long history of heart problems. She had been increasingly tired, with shortness of breath on exertion, orthopnea, and palpitations. A mitral valve replacement had been carried out 3 years previously and this had stabilized the symptoms of heart failure but was followed by episodes of atrial fibrillation, which had been particularly severe for the 6 months before admission.

Extract 4

A 64-year-old man presents to the emergency department (ED) due to an inability to urinate for the past 24 hours. In addition, he complains of an unintentional weight loss of 20 lb over the past 6 months, night sweats, and fatigue. On examination, he is thin and in moderate distress. His blood pressure is 168/92 mmHg, heart rate is 102 beats per minute, temperature is 37. 7 ℃, and respiratory rate is 22 breaths per minute. The abdominal examination reveals a tenderness mass in the suprapubic area. On rectal examination, the prostate is firm, nontender, and somewhat irregular.

Extract 5

On examination, he looked unwell. His pulse rate was 100/minute. He had a palpable spleen. The combination of fever and rigors in a patient who has recently returned from Africa strongly suggests a diagnosis of malaria. The incubation period is usually 10-14 days. In this case, the patient admitted he had not been taking prophylaxis regularly. The diagnosis was confirmed by the presence of parasites in his blood film.

Now you'll hear Part One again. This is the end of Part One. Now look at Part Two.
You will hear a conversation between a chief physician and a patient. For each of the following statements, decide whether it is True (A) or False (B). If there is not enough information to answer True (A) or False (B), choose Not Given (C). Mark the corresponding letter on your answer sheet. You will hear the recording twice.

Chief Physician: How are you today, sir?
Patient: Not bad, professor. But the pain still bothers me much.
Chief Physician: Oh. Could you point the positions of the pain?
Patient: Of course. Mainly in my waist, as well as the chest, back and thigh.
Chief Physician: Always such painful?
Patient: No. At the beginning, it didn't reach such a large range and mainly appeared after activities although resulting in the operation 14 years ago. I did feel much better after it. But during recent years, the pain is always

torturing me so much that I can hardly turn around and have to use great efforts for each sitting-down or standing-up.

Chief Physician: Anything else uncomfortable?

Patient: Yes. My appetite has become less and less in recent years. However, I often feel hungry, which sometimes causes rapid heartbeat and sweating. So I have to eat something to relieve it, but you see, I can only eat a little, otherwise, I will feel abdominal distention, and gastric pain sometimes.

Chief Physician: Oh, gastric pain. What time do you feel it more significant? Will you get better after meals?

Patient: Oh, it's irregular. Whether I'm empty or full, it may come, and sometimes it wakes me up during midnight.

Chief Physician: And anything else?

Patient: Oh, I'm always feeling weakness and exhausted.

Chief Physician: Do your bowels and urine always go well?

Patient: Er ... No. In fact I have been always constipated and piss much at night.

Chief Physician: Are you coughing recently?

Patient: No.

Chief Physician: Any changes in your body weight?

Patient: Yes. I have been always becoming thinner these years. Now I have lost over 10 kg.

Chief Physician: Do you know yourself in the emergency room 4 days ago?

Patient: Yes. But at that time I was quite confused, just feeling thirsty and longing for water, while nausea and vomiting at the same time. I recognized here on recovering awareness.

Chief Physician: All right. Now could we give you an examination?

Patient: Of course.

Now you'll hear Part Two again. This is the end of Part Two. Now look at Part Three. You will hear a conversation between the patient Krista and the nurse Shirley about her concerns on Cesarean section. For questions 14—20, choose the most appropriate answer. Mark the corresponding letter on your answer sheet. You will hear the conversation twice.

Krista: Hi, Shirley, I am scheduled to have a C-section at 9 am next Monday. May I ask you some questions?

Shirley: Sure, please.

Krista: What kind of anesthesia will I have for the Cesarean?

Shirley: You are going to have epidural anesthesia.

Krista: I am not going to be put to sleep, right?

Shirley: You're right. With an epidural, you will be awake and alert. Once the baby is out of your uterus, the doctor probably will let you see the baby, and if you want, you can hold your baby for a while.

Krista: Good, that's what I hope to do. My husband will be allowed to stay in the operating room, won't he?

Shirley: Yes. On the scheduled day, you come here with your husband. The nurse will prepare you first and transport you to the OR. When everything is ready and it's time for the operation, your husband will be called in to sit by you.

Krista: Will the operation scare him?

Shirley: The seat for your husband to sit in will be behind a screen. He will not be able to see the operation.

Krista: Why should he sit behind the screen?

Shirley: Because his role in the OR is to support you. He is not there to observe the operation, does that make sense?

Krista: Yes, it does.

Shirley: It is not recommended that a lay person watch the operation. We have had husbands passed out in the delivery suite.

Krista: I am also worried about that. OK, I'll tell my husband he won't get to watch the operation. But he can hold the baby, right?

Shirley: Sure he can. He is there for you and the baby as well.

Krista: What about recovery after the Cesarean?

Shirley: After the surgical procedure is done, you will be sent to the PACU, the post anesthesia care unit. You are going to stay there for a few hours until your vital signs are stable.

Krista: Will the baby go with me to the PACU?

Shirley: No. Usually the baby will be sent to the nursery, where the nurse will give him or her a bath and administer some required medications. A pediatrician might come to see the baby during that period of time.

Krista: That's good.

Shirley: When the anesthesiologist signs you off, you will be transferred to the postpartum unit.

Krista: Will I be able to breastfeed after a C-section?

Shirley: Yes, actually, breastfeeding is encouraged. You can start breastfeeding right away after the surgery although you might not have any milk produced.

Krista: I learned this from a book. The baby's suction will stimulate milk production and it's good for uterine recovery.

Shirley: You're right.

Krista: I'll try to breastfeed my baby.

Shirley: That's good for you and your baby.

Krista： Thank you for answering my questions.

Shirley： It's my pleasure.

Now you'll hear Part Three again. This is the end of Part Three. Now look at Part Four. You will hear a talk of case history about a patient Mr. Zhang. Complete the notes. In each Blank, write only one word. Write the answers on your answer sheet. You will hear the talk twice.

Male： Zhang Hang, a 45-year-old man of oversea Chinese, presented in September 14, 2017 with lethargy and polyuria. His family physicians had noted a high serum calcium (3.4 mmol/L) and a low albumin (30 g/L). Twenty years ago, just two years after he had immigrated to Canada, he had undergone an emergency portacaval shunt for bleeding esophageal varices. On that occasion, but on no other, he had received blood transfusions. He routinely drank two glasses of wine with his evening meal. There were no other risk factors for liver disease known. In the interval, he had been well and had required medical attention. The referring specialist had assayed the parathyroid hormone (PTH) level at 21.6 pmol/L (normal 0—5.8 pmol/L). A search for a parathyroid adenoma or metastatic cancer was undertaken. Ultrasound examination of the abdomen revealed a solitary lesion in the right lobe of the liver. CT scan of the neck and the bone scan were normal. Initial treatment consisted of intravenous rehydration and diuretics. Subsequently, the patient felt much better.

On examination, the patient has a fit looking, with considerable anxiety regarding the state of his health and his prognosis, with no evidence of confusion or amnesia. Signs of liver disease included scattered spider nevi on his chest. He did not appear jaundiced or anemic. No lymphadenopathy was palpable. There was no ankle edema. His abdomen was soft, with no organomegaly or ascites.

The dynamic CT scan showed a middle (3 cm×3 cm) solid occupied lesion in anatomic right lobe of the liver. Doppler ultrasound of the liver vessels confirmed the presence of a side to side portacaval shunt with blood flow in the portal vein away from the liver. There were no retroperitoneal varices and the spleen was of normal size.

Now you'll hear Part Four again. This is the end of Part Four. You now have five minutes to write your answers on the answer sheet. You have one more minute. This is the end of the test.

参考答案与试题评析

I Listening

Part One

第一部分是信息配对题,考生在听完每一个病例描述后,需要选出正确的对该病例的概述。

1.【语段大意】本题中的患者是一位 55 岁的家庭主妇,主诉是疲劳和不适。否认进食增多但体重增加,有便秘及脱发等症状。

【解题思路】C 听到 tiredness/fatigue, malaise, weight gain, constipation, hair loss 等这些词。很显然,答案为 C。

2.【语段大意】本题中的患者是一位 48 岁的男性,咽痛、发烧两天,否认咳嗽或恶心。体温 38.3 ℃,扁桃体肿大但无分泌物,双侧颈部淋巴结肿大触痛。快速链球菌抗原测定为阴性。

【解题思路】E 可听到 swollen tonsils, no exudates 故 E 为正确答案,F 为错误干扰项。

3.【语段大意】本题中的患者是一名长期患有心脏疾病的 22 岁学生,疲劳、用力后气短、端坐呼吸、心悸。三年前接受二尖瓣置换术(mitral valve replacement),心衰症状稳定,但伴有房颤发作,入院前半年尤其严重。

【解题思路】B 可听到 mitral valve replacement 故选项 B 为正确答案。

4.【语段大意】本题中的患者为一名 64 岁的男性,因 24 小时无尿来到急诊科。主诉为体重减轻、盗汗、疲劳。

【解题思路】A 可听到 inability to urinate, weight loss, night sweats and fatigue 与选项 A 吻合,故答案为 A。

5.【语段大意】本题描述的是一名刚从非洲回来的病人,他可能患上了疟疾。

【解题思路】D 可听到 having malaria。显然答案为 D。

Part Two

【语篇大意】第二部分是主任医师跟患者的对话,考生根据听到的对话内容判读正误。

6.【解题思路】B 本题是一道细节题,文中病人描述疼痛主要在腰部,还有胸部、后背及大腿,但本题中描述成腹部、胸部、后背及大腿,故答案为 B。

7.【解题思路】A 对话中病人提及 14 年前曾接受手术来缓解疼痛,故答案为 A。

8.【解题思路】B 病人描述之前的疼痛部位没有这么广,主要是在活动后出现。本题关于疼痛范围的描述有误,所以答案为 B。

9.【解题思路】A 近几年,病人苦受疼痛折磨,几乎不能转身,每次坐下或站起都很费劲,题目中的描述完全吻合,故 A 正确。

10.【解题思路】B 在询问病史时,病人提及食欲不佳,但常有饥饿感,并且一饿就觉得心慌、出冷汗。题目中描述病人有饱胀感、食欲不佳,与原文不符,因此选 B。

11.【解题思路】C 整篇对话并没有提到病人多次去看医生,但病情并无好转,故选 C。

12.【解题思路】B 病人主诉包括疲劳、无力、便秘、夜尿但无咳嗽,故选 B。

13.【解题思路】A 对话中提到四天前,病人意识模糊,进入急救室,故 A 正确。

Part Three

【语篇大意】第三部分是一位即将进行剖宫产手术的产妇(Krista)向护士(Shirley)咨询剖宫产的相关问题,要求考生在理解的基础上完成七道选择题。

14.【解题思路】C 本题问 Krista 剖宫产的时间,对话开始明确提到是 9 am next Monday,所以答案很显然是 C。关键信息:I am scheduled to have a C-section at 9 am next Monday.

15.【解题思路】B 本题是 Krista 向 Shirley 咨询的第一个问题,即本次剖宫产中会采用何种麻醉。护士明确回答是硬膜外麻醉(epidural anesthesia),故 B 为正确答案。关键信息:What kind of anesthesia will I have for the Cesarean? /You are going to have epidural anesthesia.

16.【解题思路】C 本题还是跟麻醉有关的问题,硬膜外麻醉时,产妇是清醒的,故答案为 C。关键信息:You're right. With an epidural, you will be awake and alert.

17.【解题思路】A 产妇丈夫在手术室中是坐在屏幕后的,因为他的主要任务不是观摩手术过程,也不是去抱孩子,而是给产妇提供支持。所以答案应该选 A。关键信息:Because his role in the OR is to support you. He is not there to observe the operation, does that make sense? /The seat for your husband to sit in will be behind a screen. He will not be able to see the operation.

18.【解题思路】B 剖宫产手术后,病人从产房(delivery suite)出来,首先会被送到麻醉后监护室(PACU),等麻醉清醒后才会送到产后恢复室(postpartum unit),所以本题答案为 B。关键信息:After the surgical procedure is done, you will be sent to the PACU, the post anesthesia care unit.

19.【解题思路】A 麻醉师同意离开后,产妇应该转入产后恢复室(postpartum unit),所以本题答案为 A。关键信息:When the anesthesiologist signs you off, you will be transferred to the postpartum unit.

20.【解题思路】A 本题涉及 Krista 问的最后一个问题,剖宫产后是否能够母乳喂养。事实上,我们提倡母乳喂养,剖宫产后尽管不能立刻产奶但也可以开始母乳喂养,婴儿的吮吸能刺激乳汁的分泌,对于子宫的恢复也是有帮助的。显然只有 A 是错误的,B 和 C 都是正确的。本题答案为 A。关键信息:You can start breastfeeding right away after the surgery although you might not have any milk produced. The baby's suction will stimulate milk production and it's good for uterine recovery.

Part Four

【语篇大意】第四部分是一段病历描述,在听完后需要完成表格中的五个信息填空。如果考生对病历书写的格式以及内容比较熟悉的话,这一部分就相对容易了。

【解题思路】

21. albumin 文中提到家庭医生发现病人高血钙、低白蛋白。此处应填 albumin.

22. varices 文中提到既往史部分提到病人 20 年前因食管静脉曲张出血而做了急诊门腔静脉分流术,此处应填 varices.

23. solitary 文中提到腹部超声检查发现右肝叶有单个肿块,根据短文内容,此处应填 solitary。

24. occupied 文中讲述动态 CT 扫描显示右肝叶有中等大小的实质性占位病变(solid occupied lesion),故此处应填 occupied。

25. diuretics 文中讲述最初治疗包括静脉补液和给予利尿剂(diuretics),此处应填 diuretics。

II Reading

Part One

【文章大意】文章指出神经递质和一些化学物质是主导人类睡眠的重要因素,同时介绍了夜间睡眠的五个阶段及各个阶段中的身体状态。

【解题思路】

26. B 参照第一段最后一句话"Moreover, sleep affects our daily functioning and our physical and mental health in many ways that we are just beginning to understand."。

27. D 参照第二段第一句话"Nerve-signaling chemicals called neurotransmitters control whether we are asleep or awake by acting on different groups of nerve cells, or neurons, in the brain.",第二段其余部分举出脑干神经元、大脑基部神经元以及腺苷控制睡眠的例子。

28. F 参照第三段第一句"During sleep, we usually pass through five phases of sleep: stages 1, 2, 3, 4, and REM (rapid eye movement) sleep."。

29. A 参照第四段"During stage 1 ... When we enter stage 2 sleep ... In stage 3 ... By stage 4 ..."。

30. E 参照第五段 "When we switch into REM sleep, our breathing ... our eyes ... and our limb muscles ... Our heart rate ... "。

31. D 定位第三段第二句话"These stages progress in a cycle from stage 1 to REM sleep, then the cycle starts over again with stage 1."。

32. A 定位第二段第一句话"Nerve-signaling chemicals called neurotransmitters control whether we are asleep or awake by acting on different groups of nerve cells, or neurons, in the brain."。

33. F 定位第三段第三句话"We spend almost 50 percent of our total sleep time in stage 2 sleep ... "和第四段第六句话"When we enter stage 2 sleep, our eye movements stop and our brain waves become slower ... "。

34. B 定位第四段第九和第十二句话"It is very difficult to wake someone during stages 3 and 4, which together are called deep sleep. Some children experience bedwetting, night terrors, or sleepwalking during deep sleep."。

35. E 定位第五段最后一句话"When people awaken during REM sleep, they often describe bizarre and illogical tales—dreams."。

Part Two

【文章大意】文章主要介绍了肠道易激综合征的症状、发病机制以及诱因等内容。

【解题思路】

36．D　参照第一段第一句话"Irritable bowel syndrome（IBS）is a common intestinal condition characterized by abdominal pain and cramps；changes in bowel movements（diarrhea，constipation，or both）…"。

37．C　参照第二段第一句话。

38．A　参照第三段第二句话"It is called a functional disorder because it is thought to result from changes in the activity of the major part of the large intestine（the colon）."。B和C选项意为形态上紊乱和结构上的改变，不符合原文。

39．B　参照第三段第九句话"Sometimes there is too little peristalsis，which can slow the passage of undigested material through the colon and cause constipation."。

40．C　第四段第一句话"Some kinds of food and drink appear to play a key role in triggering IBS attacks."指出一些食品和饮料是IBS的重要诱因，接着下句以巧克力、奶制品、咖啡因及大量酒精为例说明了这个问题，显然答案为C选项，意为致病因素。

41．D　文章第四段第一句话、第五段第一句和最后一句话提到了一些食物和饮料、压力及某些激素是IBS的诱因，而从第五段第二句话"Although researchers do not yet understand all of the links between changes in the nervous system and IBS，they point out the similarities between mild digestive upsets and IBS."中看出，轻度消化不良与肠道易激综合征具有相似性，而不是肠道易激综合征的原因，因而选D。

42．C　根据第三段第八句话"In IBS，however，the normal rhythm and intensity of peristalsis is disrupted."判断C选项正确；根据第二段第三句话"Although modern medicine recognizes that stress can trigger IBS attacks，medical specialists agree that IBS is a genuine physical disorder…"判断B选项错误；根据第四段最后一句话"Characteristically，IBS symptoms rarely occur at night and disrupt the patient's sleep."判断D选项错误；而A选项未提及，因而本题选C。

Part Three

【文章大意】本文介绍了病毒抗癌疗法的优点、抗癌机制及相关研究成果。

【解题思路】

43．B　根据第二段"If successful，virus therapy could eventually form a third pillar alongside radiotherapy and chemotherapy in the standard arsenal against cancer，while avoiding some of the debilitating side-effects."可以看出，病毒疗法可避免导致患者身体虚弱的某些副作用，而不是完全没有副作用。

44．A　参照第三段最后一句话"Cancer Research UK said yesterday that it was exciting by the potential of Prof Seymour's pioneering techniques."。

45．C　病毒能够杀死癌细胞在文章前几段得到多次表述，而病毒能够抑制癌细胞再生在文中未提及。

46．A　参照第五段第三、四句话"If you can get a virus into a tumor，viruses find them a very good place to be because there's no immune system to stop them replicating. You can regard it as the cancer's Achilles' heel."。

47．B　参照第六段第一句话"Only a small amount of the virus needs to get to the cancer."。

48. A 参照文章第七段。

49. C 题干在文中未提及。

50. A 参照第十段"'What we've done is make chemical modifications to the virus to put a polymer coat around it—it's a stealth virus when you inject it,' he said."。本段承接上一段,因此,"he"指代"Prof Seymour"。

Part Four

【文章大意】文章介绍了人被挠痒时发笑的原因,大笑对身体和健康的影响以及大笑时人脑活动状态。

【解题思路】

51. A 上几句中"but the inevitable occurs:what you anticipated—you are tickled and in hysterics you chuckle, titter, and burst into uncontrollable laughter."指出人被挠痒会咯咯笑,下段"Tickling is caused by a light sensation across our skin."分析了这种现象的原因,因而 A 是合理衔接。

52. C 上句提到"Heavy laughter is caused by someone or something placing repeated pressure on a person and tickling a particular area.",在身体某个地方挠痒时会发出大笑,C 选项紧接着列举具体部位。

53. E 本段谈到"Laughter requires the coordination of many muscles throughout the body. Laughter also increases blood pressure and heart rate, changes breathing, reduces levels of certain neurochemicals (catecholamines, hormones) and provides a boost to the immune system."。大笑需要身体各部位肌肉的协调,会影响身体诸多健康指标,对健康也有促进作用,因而作为本段首句,E 是合理衔接。

54. B 参照第四段第三句话"Preliminary results indicate that the humor-processing pathway includes parts of the frontal lobe brain area, important for cognitive processing; the supplementary motor area, important for movement; and the nucleus accumbens, associated with pleasure."。

55. F 在上文"Investigations support the notion that parts of the frontal lobe are involved in humor. Subjects' brains were imaged while they listened to jokes."谈及的实验中得到证实,前额叶部分区域参与了幽默信息处理过程。当受试者在听笑话时,他们大脑活动的成像表明只有他们觉得这个笑话很好笑时,前额叶的部分区域才会受到激发,F 是合理衔接。

Part Five

【文章大意】文章介绍了磁疗的原理、副作用以及外界对这种疗法的态度。

【解题思路】

56. A 此处意为很多具有磁性的用品被认为有治疗功能,与上句中"therapy"相呼应。

57. B 此处意为广告宣称这些用品可以治疗百病,尤其是疼痛。

58. C 此处意为这些产品的治疗原理是平衡人体的电能,principle 的意思是"原理""准则"等。

59. D 此处意为这些产品可以缓解疼痛,最主要的是肌肉和关节疼痛,"primarily"一词与"occasionally"形成对照。

60. C 此处意为磁性用品可以用在身体的诸多部位,因此用"among"。

61. B 此处意为坚持磁疗的人认为只要患者处在磁场中,磁力疗法就可以治愈病痛。"be exposed to"意思是"暴露于"。

62. A 此处意为世卫组织声称少量磁能对人体无伤害。

63. B 此处意为装有起搏器、准备做磁共振或进行放射治疗的病患应避免磁力,这是因为这些医疗设备会受到磁力干扰。这里 as 表示原因。

64. C "关于……的研究"用"study on ... "。

65. D 此处意为绝大多数的病人在进行磁疗后感觉疼痛减轻,"significant"表示"显著的"。

Ⅲ Writing

66.【范文】

Should Induced Abortion Be Controlled?

For a long time, there has been a common phenomenon of women taking induced abortion. But, in my opinion, induced abortion has many negative effects. First of all, the great pain and huge loss of blood in induced abortion will certainly affect women's health. It usually takes at least one week for them to recover. In addition, women who have had several abortions may suffer from spontaneous abortion and, as a result, may lose the right to be mothers.

Abortion is inhumane. In most cases, women are forced to have abortions, so, to some extent, abortion is a kind of murder in disguise. Also, abortion provides excuses for irresponsible sex. Many abortion cases are the result of indecent sexual relationships and may damage public morality.

So, we should control abortion, and only under certain necessary circumstances (e. g. deformed embryo) should we take abortion so as to protect women's rights and ensure the good health of our children, creating a harmonious society. (161 words)

【审题】

本部分给出段落提示句,要求考生从健康和人道这两个方面分析人工流产,然后阐明自己的观点。注意第三部分的结论要与前面的分析前后呼应,符合逻辑。文章属说明文,除遵守说明文写作的基本要求外,写作中的一个重点和难点是如何正确写出一些涉及医疗卫生领域话题的英语表达,如"人工流产、自然流产"等。

【范文评析】

首先根据作文任务给定的信息,指出目前存在的一种社会现象,点明文章的主题。文章的重点放在人工流产的危害分析上:第一段第二句总领全文,随后从两个方面进行论述。一方面是对女性身体造成伤害,另一方面讲述人工流产是不人道的。第三段简明扼要,进行总结,指出我们应该禁止人工流产。

整篇文章段落清晰,能恰当的表明主题,阐述部分充实有序,每个主题句都有适当的扩展或说明;In addition, In most cases, Also 等词语较好地衔接文章;倒装结构的使用(we should control abortion, and only under certain necessary circumstances (e. g. deformed embryo) should we take abortion so as to protect women's rights and ensure the good health of our children, creating a harmonious society.)是文章比较精彩的地方。

医护英语水平考试(三级)
模拟训练(四)

听力文本

This is METS-3 listening test. There are four parts in the test, Part One, Two, Three, and Four. You will hear each part twice. We will now stop for a moment before we start the test. Please ask any questions because you must not speak during the test. Now, look at the instructions for Part One.

You will hear five extracts from conversations taking place in different clinical departments. Choose which case each doctor is discussing from the list A—F. Use each letter A—F only once. There is one extra letter which you do not need to use. Mark the corresponding letter on your answer sheet. You will hear each extract twice. Now we are ready to start.

Extract 1

Preoperative radio-graphs show a non-displaced right intertrochanteric fracture. That is why you have excruciating pain in your right leg. Your right leg has been externally rotated, slightly shorter than your left leg, and adducted. Intraoperatively, you will be given spinal anesthesia and positioned on an orthopedic table with your right hip abducted and secured in traction.

Extract 2

You have been in remission for 14 months from aggressively treated ovarian carcinoma. It is common that you have mild abdominal distention and tenderness on deep palpation of the lower pelvis. It is reported that you claimed a feeling of fullness in the lower abdomen, loss of appetite, and inability to sleep through the night. To avoid possible recurrence or sequelae of your ovarian cancer, you'd better have a follow-up visit with your oncologist every month.

Extract 3

Your family history was significant for cardiovascular disease. Your father died at the age of 62 of an acute myocardial infarction. Your mother had bilateral carotid endarterectomies and a femoral-popliteal bypass procedure and died at the age of 72 of congestive heart failure. Your older sister died from a ruptured aortic aneurysm at the age of 65. Your ECG on admission presented tachycardia with a rate of 126 bpm with inverted T waves.

Extract 4

The results of bone marrow aspiration were positive for myelofibrosis. You need to go through a 6-month therapy regimen of iron supplements in the form of ferrous sulfate tablets and receive weekly vitamin B_{12} injections. Interferon was given every other week in addition to erythropoiesis therapy.

Extract 5

You have a history of mild asthma since age 4, with at least one attack per week. In an acute attack, you will have mild dyspnea, diffuse wheezing, yet an adequate air exchange that responds to bron-chodilators. We decide to send you to pulmonary health services for a consult with a specialist and pulmonary function studies to clear you for surgery.

Now You'll hear Part One again. This is the end of Part One. Now look at Part Two. You will hear a conversation between a reporter and a WHO official. For each of the following statements, decide whether it is True (A) or False (B). If there is not enough information to answer True (A) or False (B), choose Not Given (C). Mark the corresponding letter on your answer sheet. You will hear the recording twice.

Reporter: I am Christopher Jones Cruise. I am interviewing Douglas Bettcher who is the WHO director for the prevention of non-communicable diseases. Mr. Bettcher, the WHO says progress is being made in reducing deaths from non-communicable diseases, so what are non-communicable diseases?

WHO Official: Non-communicable diseases, or NCDs, including heart disease, stroke, cancer, diabetes and chronic lung disease, are collectively responsible for almost 70% of all deaths worldwide. Every year, 15 million adults die before they reach old age. It's noted they often die in the most productive period of their lives, between the ages of 30 and 70.

Reporter: What are their risk factors?

WHO Official: The rise of NCDs has been driven by primarily four major risk factors: tobacco use, physical inactivity, the harmful use of alcohol and unhealthy diets. The epidemic of NCDs poses devastating health consequences for individuals, families and communities, and threatens to overwhelm health systems. The socioeconomic costs associated with NCDs make the prevention and control of these diseases a major development imperative for the 21st century.

Reporter： Are premature deaths from NCDs a problem in most countries?

WHO Official： Eighty percent of the deaths are in countries that are already often stressed; their health systems are stressed with the usual—the conventional burdens of disease, communicable diseases, maternal-child health problems. And, then this is an added, extremely large burden for the health system. Costa Rica and Iran are at the top of a list of 10 countries that have been most successful at reducing deaths from non-communicable diseases. It says six countries have failed to make any progress against such deaths. Five of the six are in Africa. They are Angola, Equatorial Guinea, Guinea-Bissau, Sao Tome Principe and South Sudan. The sixth country is Micronesia in the western Pacific.

Reporter： I heard progress is being made on cutting premature death from NCDs by one-third by the year 2030, would you give us more details?

WHO Official： Of course. What you just mentioned is a Sustainable Development Goal for United Nations member countries. Increasing numbers of people— particularly children and adolescents—are suffering from obesity, overweight and diabetes. If we don't take action now to protect people from non-communicable diseases, we will condemn today's and tomorrow's youth to lives of ill-health and reduced economic opportunities. WHO's mission is to provide leadership and the evidence base for international action on surveillance, prevention and control of NCDs. Urgent government action is needed to meet global targets to reduce the burden of NCDs. By the way, early this month, WHO and Government of Denmark hosted a Global Dialogue to address the critical gap in financing for national NCD responses. The goal for the meeting was to share information on existing and potential sources of finance and development cooperation at the local, national, regional and global levels, and explore new opportunities for multistakeholder and multisectoral partnerships in order to catalyse action for effective national NCD responses.

Now you'll hear Part Two again. This is the end of Part Two. Now look at Part Three. You will hear a discussion among an instructor and two medical students. For questions 14—20, choose the most appropriate answer. Mark the corresponding letter on your answer sheet. You will hear the discussion twice.

Instructor： Today we are going to discuss double pneumonia. Who would like to speak first?

Student 1： Double pneumonia is an infection of both lungs. People who have the influenza virus infection, some types of streptococcal bacterial infections, respiratory syncytial virus or RSV, and some other infections can develop double pneumonia.

Student 2: A virus, bacteria or fungus causes the tiny sacs of the lungs, called alveoli, to become inflamed and fill with fluid or pus, causing a range of symptoms, including breathing difficulties.

Instructor: Yes. Because double pneumonia affects both lungs, a person may find it extremely difficult to breathe. It is impossible to tell if a person has pneumonia or double pneumonia based on symptoms alone so anybody who thinks they may have pneumonia must see a doctor as soon as possible. What are common symptoms for pneumonia?

Student 1: Symptoms of pneumonia include a high fever, chills, or shaking. Rarely, some people develop an unusually low temperature.

Student 2: A cough that gets worse, coughing up thick mucus or phlegm, and chest pain when coughing or breathing.

Instructor: Right. Nausea, vomiting, or diarrhea may be along with respiratory symptoms. As pneumonia progresses, it can cause serious complications — particularly in people with weakened immune systems due to age, illness, or debilitating diseases, such as HIV or AIDS. What are the complications of pneumonia?

Student 1: Sepsis, I think.

Instructor: Sepsis, yes, an infection that causes systemic inflammation in the body. It is a serious illness that can be fatal.

Student 2: Lung abscesses and pleural effusions.

Instructor: Exactly. The pleurae are two membranes that line the outside of the lungs within the chest cavity. Usually, a small amount of pleural fluid fills the gap between the membranes, but pneumonia may cause an accumulation of this fluid. If there is a buildup of fluid, or it becomes infected, a pleural effusion can cause death. Though it is a serious infection, it is treatable. Anyone that has difficulty breathing and a high fever should treat it as a medical emergency. Treatment for double pneumonia depends on what caused it and how it has affected the body.

Student 2: People who have bacterial pneumonia will need antibiotic therapy.

Instructor: Exactly! People with severe infections related to pneumonia, such as infectious pleural effusion or sepsis, will need intravenous antimicrobial therapy. People with viral pneumonia will not respond to antibiotics, which do not work to treat viral infection. Other treatments for pneumonia focus on preventing further damage to the lungs and ensuring a person can breathe. Some people may require supplemental oxygen or monitoring in a hospital setting. Rest and remaining hydrated may also help. While coughing can be unpleasant, coughing helps the body rid itself of the infection. People who have double pneumonia should not take a cough suppressant medicine unless a doctor recommends doing so.

Now you'll hear Part Three again. This is the end of Part Three. Now look at Part Four. You will hear a speech on e-cigarettes, or vaping. Complete the notes. In each blank, write only one word. Write the answers on your answer sheet. You will hear the speech twice.

Male: If you have thought about trying to kick a smoking habit, you're not alone. Nearly seven out of 10 smokers say they want to stop. Quitting smoking is one of the best things you can do for your health. Smoking harms nearly every organ in your body, including your heart. Nearly one-third of deaths from heart disease are the result of smoking and secondhand smoke.

You might be tempted to turn to electronic cigarettes as a way to ease the transition from traditional cigarettes to not smoking at all. But is smoking e-cigarettes, which is also called vaping, better for you than using tobacco products? Here are some truth you need to know about vaping.

Truth No. 1: Vaping is less harmful than traditional smoking. E-cigarettes heat nicotine flavorings and other chemicals to create water vapor that you inhale. Regular tobacco cigarettes contain 7,000 chemicals, many of which are toxic. While we don't know exactly what chemicals are in e-cigarettes, experts says "there's almost no doubt that they expose you to fewer toxic chemicals than traditional cigarettes."

Truth No. 2: Vaping is still bad for your health. Nicotine is the primary agent in both regular cigarettes and e-cigarettes, and it is highly addictive. It causes you to crave smoke and suffer withdrawal symptoms if you ignore the craving. Nicotine is also a toxic substance. It raises your blood pressure and spikes your adrenaline, which increases your heart rate and the likelihood of having a heart attack. There are many unknowns about vaping, including what chemicals make up the vapor and how they affect physical health over the long term.

Truth No. 3: Electronic cigarettes are just as addictive as traditional ones. Both e-cigarettes and regular cigarettes contain nicotine, which research suggests may be as addictive as heroin and cocaine. What's worse, many e-cigarette users get even more nicotine than they would from a tobacco product—you can buy extra-strength cartridges, which have a higher concentration of nicotine, or you can increase the e-cigarette's voltage to get a greater hit of the substance.

Truth No. 4: Electronic cigarettes aren't the best smoking cessation tool. Although they've been marketed as an aid to help you quit smoking, e-cigarettes have not received Food and Drug Administration approval as smoking cessation devices. A recent study found that most people who intended to use e-cigarettes to kick the nicotine habit ended up continuing to smoke both traditional and e-cigarettes.

Truth No. 5: A new generation is getting hooked on nicotine. Among youth, e-cigarettes are more popular than any traditional tobacco products. In 2015, the US surgeon general reported that e-cigarette use among high school students had increased by 900 percent, and 40 percent of young e-cigarette users had never smoked regular tobacco.

There's a strong link between smoking and cardiovascular disease, and between smoking and cancer. But the sooner you quit, the quicker your body can rebound and repair itself. Talk to your doctor about what smoking cessation program or tools would be best for you.

Now you'll hear Part Four again. This is the end of Part Four. You now have five minutes to write your answers on the answer sheet. You have one more minute. This is the end of the listening test.

参考答案与试题评析

Ⅰ Listening

Part One

1.【语段大意】 医生对患者右股骨粗隆间骨折术前 X 光片进行解释,阐明患者右腿疼痛的原因,包括右腿外旋、短于左腿、内收。随后,医生阐明手术将进行脊椎麻醉,对髋关节进行固定和牵引。

【解题思路】D 可听到 right intertrochanteric fracture, pain in your right leg, intraoperatively 等关键信息。

2.【语段大意】医生分析患者卵巢癌积极治疗 14 个月后的身体状况,认为轻微腹胀、下骨盆压痛、下腹部饱腹感、食欲不振、失眠等都是常见症状,建议每个月与肿瘤专家进行一次随访。

【解题思路】B 可听到 ovarian carcinoma, recurrence or sequelae of your ovarian cancer, have a follow-up visit with your oncologist 等关键信息。

3.【语段大意】患者有心血管疾病家族史。父亲死于心肌梗死,母亲死于心力衰竭,姐姐死于主动脉瘤破裂,患者入院时心电图表现为心动过速等。

【解题思路】A 可听到 family history, cardiovascular disease, acute myocardial infarction, congestive heart failure, a ruptured aortic aneurysm, tachycardia 等关键词。

4.【语段大意】骨髓穿刺结果显示患者骨髓纤维变性呈阳性。医生提供了一个 6 个月的治疗方案,建议补铁、注射维生素 B_{12}、进行促红细胞生成素疗法,并使用干扰素。

【解题思路】C 可听到 were positive for myelofibrosis, therapy regimen 等关键信息。

5.【语段大意】医生向患者阐述了其哮喘的发病情况,并告知患者,决定将患者送到肺部健康服务中心进行会诊,以便进行手术。

【解题思路】F 可听到 We decide to send you to pulmonary health services for a consult with a specialist and pulmonary function studies to clear you for surgery 这一关键句。

Part Two

【语篇大意】一位记者对一位国际卫生组织官员关于非传染性疾病的采访。

【解题思路】

6. B 官员回答中提到非传染性疾病占到世界死亡人口的 70%,故答案为 B。

7. A 官员在回答中指出,患病人群通常在一生中最富生产能力(the most productive period)的时期死亡,即 30 至 70 岁之间,故答案为 A。

8. A 官员阐述了非传染性疾病的四大致病因素:吸烟(tobacco use)、不运动(physical inactivity)、有害饮酒(the harmful use of alcohol) 和不健康饮食(unhealthy diets),所以答案为 A。

9. A 官员提到非传染性疾病的社会经济成本使得对这类疾病的防治成为 21 世纪的一项迫切任务,所以选 A。

10. C 整篇听力未提及非传染性疾病死亡与国家经济水平有关系,因此选 C。

11. B 官员提到有 6 个国家在防治非传染性疾病方面没有进步,其中有 5 个是非洲国家,所以选 B。

12. A 官员提到,世界卫生组织的任务是领导监测、预防和控制非传染性疾病,所以选 A。

13. A 听力最后部分,官员提到,本月初,世界卫生组织和丹麦政府主办了一次全球对话,以解决国家防治非传染性疾病筹资方面的严重缺口,故 A 正确。

Part Three

【语篇大意】两位医学生与老师讨论双侧肺炎的相关问题。

【解题思路】

14. A 双侧肺炎即两侧肺部感染,故答案为 A。

15. C 对话中提到病毒和细菌会导致肺泡发炎,故答案为 C。关键信息:A virus, bacteria or fungus causes the tiny sacs of the lungs, called alveoli, to become inflamed …

16. C 对话中提到肺炎的症状包括发烧、发冷或颤抖、少数人会出现体温过低、咳痰、胸痛或伴有恶心呕吐或痢疾等,所以答案应该选 C。关键信息:Symptoms of pneumonia include a high fever, chills, or shaking. Rarely, some people develop an unusually low temperature … /coughing up thick mucus or phlegm, and chest pain when coughing or breathing. /Nausea, vomiting, or diarrhea may be along with respiratory symptoms.

17. B 对话中提到双侧肺炎的并发症包括脓毒(sepsis)、肺脓肿(lung abscesses) 和胸腔积液(pleural effusions),故答案为 B。关键信息:Sepsis, yes, an infection that causes systemic inflammation in the body. /Lung abscesses and pleural effusions.

18. A 对话中提到胸膜是连接肺部外的胸腔的两层膜,B 为口腔,C 为腹腔,显然 A 正确。关键信息:The pleurae are two membranes that line the outside of the lungs within the chest cavity.

19. A 对话中提到患细菌性肺炎需抗生素治疗，B 为静脉抗菌药物治疗，C 为水疗，故答案为 A。关键信息：People who have bacterial pneumonia will need antibiotic therapy.

20. C 对话中提到咳嗽可能是不舒服的，故 A 项正确；咳嗽可帮助身体摆脱疾病，故 B 项正确；若非医生建议，双肺炎患者不宜服用止咳药，故答案为 C。关键信息：While coughing can be unpleasant，coughing helps the body rid itself of the infection. People who have double pneumonia should not take a cough suppressant medicine unless a doctor recommends doing so.

Part Four

【语篇大意】关于电子烟的一段讲座。

【解题思路】

21. toxic 此处为讲座中提到的关于电子烟的第一个真相，即电子烟的危害小于传统烟。电子烟加热尼古丁调味品和其他化学物质，产生让使用者可以吸入的水蒸气。普通烟草香烟含有 7 000 种化学物质，其中许多是有毒的。虽然我们不知道电子烟中到底含有什么化学物质，但专家们说："几乎毫无疑问，电子烟让使用者吸入的有毒物质少于传统香烟。"所以此处应填 toxic。

22. agent 此处为讲座中提到的关于电子烟的第二个真相，即吸电子烟仍然有害健康，因为尼古丁仍然是电子烟的主要成分。所以此处应填 agent，agent 在此处是药剂的意思。

23. concentration 此处为讲座中提到的关于电子烟的第三个真相，即吸电子烟仍然会上瘾。听力中提到，许多电子烟使用者可能摄入更多的尼古丁，因为他们可以购买额外强度的烟盒，而这些烟盒含有更高浓度的尼古丁；他们也可以通过增加电子烟的电压以获得更多的尼古丁。所以此处应填 concentration，concentration 在此处是浓度的意思。

24. cessation 此处为讲座中提到的关于电子烟的第四个真相，即电子烟不是戒烟的最好工具。听力中提到，电子烟还没有被食品和药物管理局批准为戒烟装置。所以此处应填 cessation。

25. popular 此处为讲座中提到的关于电子烟的第五个真相，即新一代对尼古丁上瘾。听力中提到，电子烟在年轻人中比普通烟草香烟更受欢迎。故此处应填 popular。

Ⅱ Reading

Part One

【文章大意】文章指出女性的饮食(比如水果和快餐)对怀孕的影响，并给出了一些饮食帮助怀孕的建议。

【解题思路】

26. C 第一段第一句"Women may be harming their chances of getting pregnant because they're avoiding fruit，or eating too much junk food."点出本文讨论的主题，即 fruit 和 junk food 两类食品(food group)对女性受孕的影响。因此选择 C。

27. A 第二段段首提出"Junk food consumption was also analyzed"之后提到，"and women who rarely ate fast food got pregnant a month quicker，on average than women

who ate fast food four times a week or more. "即很少吃快餐的女性怀孕时间要比每周吃四次或更多快餐的女性平均要快一个月。因而匹配 A 选项。

28．E 第三段第一句后半句"... keeping a healthy weight and diet is a key way to improve chances"是本段的主题句，后面句子引出的 5,598 名参与调查的女性以及第四段的内容都证明保持健康饮食（eating more fruit, minimizing fast food consumption）是提高受孕的最佳途径。因此选择 E。

29．D 第四段都是在描述杂志 Human Reproduction 对 5,598 名怀孕女性在做第一次产检时参与的调查结果和数据，并得出相应结论。因此选择 D。

30．B 第五段第一句"This study demonstrates that fruit consumption is not only safe, but beneficial for most women to optimize their fertility. "意指这项研究表明，水果的摄入不仅是安全的，而且对大多数妇女来说有利于提高她们的生育能力。因此匹配到选项 B。

31．D 定位第一段最后一句话。

32．A 定位第二段第一句。

33．E 定位第三段第二句。

34．C 定位第四段倒数第三句。

35．F 定位第五段第二句。

Part Two

【文章大意】主要报导了近 50 万女性错过 NHS 癌症筛查这一事件，并对 NHS 乳腺癌筛查进行了介绍。

【解题思路】

36．C 根据第二段第一句"has apologized for the glitch which meant 450,000 women were never sent letters inviting them to routine breast cancer checkups. "。

37．B 第四段第一句"Women aged 50 to 70 are invited for an X-ray mammogram every three years to detect any lumps or abnormalities that could be or become breast cancer."年龄在 50 岁至 70 岁的女性每三年被邀请做一次乳房射线 X 光检查，以发现任何可能成为乳腺癌的肿块或异常，故选 B。

38．A 文章第六段介绍了"Around 2.5 million women are invited to breast screening each year. In 2016/17 just 70 percent took up screening—a record low—and 18,400 cancers were picked up"（每年约有 250 万妇女接受乳房检查。在 2016/17 年，只有 70% 的人接受了筛查——这一比例创历史新低——18 400 例癌症被确诊），选 A。

39．D 第九段第一句话中的 contest 的意思就是 question，即批评家们质疑筛查给妇女带来的伤害。

40．A 第十一段第一句"In a statement today, Mr. Hunt announced the 'best estimate' is that between 135 and 270 women 'had their lives shortened as a result'"指出在今天的一份声明中，亨特先生宣布了"最好的估计"，即 135 到 270 名女性"因此而缩短了生命"。由此得出选 A。

41．B 根据文章"309,000 women are believed to still be alive and will receive a letter by the end of May telling them they may have missed screening and inviting them for a checkup now"(据信有 309 000 名女性仍然活着,她们将在 5 月底收到一封信,信中告诉她们可能错过了筛查,并邀请她们现在就去做检查),因而 A、C、D 均为错误选项。

42. C 从"In addition, and as soon as possible we will make our best endeavor to contact the next of kin of those we believe have missed a scan and subsequently died of breast cancer,"和"As well as apologizing to families affected, we wish to offer any further advice they might find helpful including ... and compensation is therefore payable."可以判断 C 选项正确。

Part Three

【文章大意】"三手烟"可能对身体造成危害。

【解题思路】

43. A 题目意思是美国研究人员发现,烟草烟雾中有害化学物质会附着在衣服、家具和地毯表面上,对人类健康造成潜在危害,此信息在文章中的第二段中出现"US researchers found that potentially harmful chemicals from tobacco smoke get trapped in clothes, furniture and carpets",故题目正确。

44. C 文章没有提及题干内容,故选项选 C。

45. B 根据第二段后半句"but can become airborne again and be circulated through office blocks, schools or other nominally smoke-free buildings.",但可以再次在空中传播,并在办公大楼、学校或其他通常禁烟建筑中传播。因此题目错误。

46. A 根据第五段"Experts said this could also be a concern for babies in the homes of smokers who are lying on furniture or carpets where these particles may have settled",题目正确。

47. B 根据第六段"this later interacts with nitrous acid formed from the gas nitrous oxide, which is released by car exhausts and gas appliances.",附着于门上的尼古丁残留物之后与亚硝酸发生反应,亚硝酸由汽车尾气和燃气用具排放出来的一氧化二氮气体形成。所以题目错误。

48. C 文章全文无提及,所以选 C。

49. B 第九段"This could also occur in electronic cigarettes, which also contain nicotine and are used in indoor public spaces much more frequently than conventional cigarettes, the authors said.",电子香烟也可能引发上述情况,电子香烟也含有尼古丁,并且在室内公共场所使用频率比传统香烟更高,故选 B。

50. A 根据第十二段"为进一步发掘研究结果,研究人员用密封容器进行了实验室试验",根据这句话得知题目正确。

Part Four

【文章大意】工作压力应作为安全隐患加以监管。

【解题思路】

51. E 第一段第二句为段落主题句,今日公布的一项针对 4,600 多名英国成年人的调查数据显示,在过去一年里,有四分之三的英国成年人因为压力过大而感到不堪重负或无力应对——尽管这一比例在女性中为 81%。根据一份关于英国心理健康和不断增加的压力流行报告,英国有三分之一的人曾有过自杀的念头,E 从而为合理选项。有助于正确选题的重要词句包括:lead to more serious mental health problems/and the MHF report found evidence of this。

52. A 第二段第二句"Thirty-two percent of adults said they had experienced suicidal feelings as a result of stress, while 16 percent of adults said they had self-harmed as a result of stress—with women and younger adults most likely to be affected. ",谈到 32％的成年人说他们因为压力而有过自杀的念头,而有 16％的成年人说他们因为压力而自我伤害——女性和年轻的成年人很可能会受到影响。A 选项接着指出就在一周前,格拉斯哥大学的研究发现,苏格兰 18 岁至 34 岁的年轻人中有九分之一曾试图自杀。

53. D 第三段中介绍"我们目前对心理危害的态度和行为不一样。MHF 表示,这些心理危害是精神健康的压力源,它压倒了包括休息、按时离开以及安全工作能力在内的各种应对机制。MHF 还呼吁应保证护士、教师、警察和其他公共部门工作人员即使在面临预算削减和员工短缺的情况下,也应有"至少两天精神健康日"。D 选项指出"压力和心理健康是旷工的第四大常见原因,但有一半的员工在感到压力太大而不愿去工作时会编造其他借口"。

54. F 第五段谈及压力引发心理健康问题和身体疾病。F 选项在首句作为概括全段的主题句最为合理。内容和信息相关。重要词句:It is also linked to physical health problems/insomnia and digestive problem/this is great information。

55. C "这包括在工作中实施心理健康计划,增强意识,监测健康和幸福",是对具体措施的描述。重要词汇:as set out in the recent independent review into/new standards/by the prime minister。

Part Five

【文章大意】文章介绍科学家发现了控制皮肤晒黑或灼伤的基因。

【解题思路】

56. A laid:铺设,其他几个选项表达不准确。

57. C affected:影响,其他几个选项表达不准确。

58. B 此处应填副词,根据"Darker-skinned people are"表示"深色皮肤的人"。usually:通常;ordinarily:通常;naturally:自然。

59. A 本句句意为:"但科学家的研究表明,除了自然的肤色之外,还有其他的遗传因素",故选 A。secure:安全 protect:保护。

60. D 此句句意为:有相同色素沉着的人也会有所不同。根据词形变异应选 variability。

61. B undertake 此处意为:这项研究使用了大量来自英国生物银行的基因数据。根据意思选 B 符合语句逻辑。

62. C 此处意为:Falchi 博士和他的同事获得了数以万计的欧洲血统的人的基因信息,这些人自称有晒黑或晒伤的倾向。选 C 符合语句逻辑。

63. A looking at 此处意为:这一发现证实了之前关于晒黑和晒伤基因基础的研究。looking at:查找;looking for:寻找;looking into:调查;looking out:调查

64. D solve 此处意为:然而,他指出,晒伤的问题不需要基因测试就可以解决。involve:包含;solve:解决

65. B avoided 此处意为:根据英国癌症研究中心(Cancer Research UK)的数据,几乎90%的黑色素瘤(皮肤癌中最严重的一种)患者可"安全地享受阳光,避免使用日光浴床"。

III Writing

66. 【范文】

How to Become a Qualified Doctor

In general, it is widely accepted that doctors' social responsibility is to save lives and heal the wounded. So what defines a qualified doctor? From my perspective, to become a respectful doctor recognized by the public, the practitioner should be both benevolent and highly skilled.

First, a respectful doctor must remain benevolent. This is because doctors are often confronted with disease and death, and their attitudes to life often have an important impact on patients. Only with benevolence will doctors try their best in the work without complaining. Though sometimes there exists misunderstanding, a qualified doctor should patiently and kindly ease the tension of doctor-patient relationship.

Second, a qualified doctor must master updated skills. In order to give patients the best treatment, doctors should constantly absorb new knowledge instead of practicing in a single way. For example, at present, there are as many as 52 treatments for breast cancer. Doctors should no longer just remove the breast. Therefore, a qualified doctor must keep learning. He or she should always focus on new medical discoveries in his/her research field, and try to find out every opportunity to keep up with the latest progress and practice.

So, to become a qualified doctor, one should remain benevolent and improve himself/herself all the time. (210 words)

【审题】

写作部分要求写一篇说明文,阐述一个合格医生应该具备的素质。文章应遵守说明文写作的基本要求,逐条清楚论述好医生应具备的素质,并通过具体细节论证自己的观点。

【范文评析】

文章第一段根据题目内容,首先陈述了医生的社会职责,随后通过提问的方式明确文章主题,并给出自己的观点。第二段首句提出分论点,随后通过因果分析和举例论证支持分论点。第三段首句总领全段,通过具体例证展开。

文章观点明确,层次清晰,段落展开充分,熟练使用提问、first、second 和 this is because、in order to 等衔接手段;倒装结构的使用(Only with benevolence will doctors try their best in the work without complaining.)则是本文句子水平上的一个亮点。

医护英语水平考试(三级)
模拟训练(五)

听力文本

This is METS-3 listening test. There are four parts in the test, Part One, Two, Three, and Four. You will hear each part twice. We will now stop for a moment before we start the test. Please ask any questions now because you must not speak during the test. Now, look at the instructions for Part One.

You will hear five extracts from conversations taking place in different clinical departments. Choose which case each doctor is discussing from the list A—F. Use each letter A—F only once. There is one extra letter which you do not need to use. Mark the corresponding letter on your answer sheet. You will hear each extract twice. Now we are ready to start.

Extract 1

I have read the report that you were admitted to the pulmonary unit with chest pain on inspiration, dyspnea, and diaphoresis. You know smoking is bad for health and smoking 1/2 packs of cigarettes per day is really too much for a 52-year-old. In addition, you were treated for primary giant cell sarcoma of the left lung 3 years ago with a lobectomy of the left lung followed by radiation and chemotherapy. Quitting smoking is really necessary.

Extract 2

I am sorry that your mother is in the ICU in the terminal stage of multisystem organ failure. She has a 20-year history of COPD. She is not conscious and is unable to breathe on her own. Her ABGs are abnormal, and she has been diagnosed with refractory ARDS. I suggest a permanent tracheostomy and family consideration of continuing or withdrawing life support.

Extract 3

Your examination on admission shows rebound tenderness in the RUQ with a positive Murphy sign. Your skin, nails, and conjunctivae are yellowish and your leukocyte count is 16,000. An ERCP and ultrasound of the abdomen suggest many small stones in your gallbladder and possibly the common bile duct. Your diagnosis is cholecystitis with cholelithiasis.

Extract 4

The previous barium enema shows some irregularities in the sigmoid and rectal segments of your large bowel. Stool samples for culture, ova, and parasites are negative. Your tentative diagnosis is irritable bowel syndrome. You should follow a lactose-free, low-residue diet and take Imodium to reduce intestinal motility. I recommend a colonoscopy.

Extract 5

It is said that you were admitted to the in-patient unit from the ER with severe right flank pain unresponsive to analgesics. And your pain did not decrease with administration of 100 mg of IV meperidine. It is also said that you had a 3-month history of chronic UTI. The problem may be caused by the calcium supplements for low bone density you were prescribed six months ago.

Now you'll hear Part One again. This is the end of Part One. Now look at Part Two.
You will hear a conversation between a reporter and a cardiologist. For each of the following statements, decide whether it is True (A) or False (B). If there is not enough information to answer True (A) or False (B), choose Not Given (C). Mark the corresponding letter on your answer sheet. You will hear the recording twice.

Reporter: I am Alice Austin. According to the American Heart Association, sedentary jobs have increased 83 percent since 1950. Physically active jobs now make up less than 20 percent of the US workforce. All of that inactivity is taking a toll on health. I am interviewing Johns Hopkins cardiologist Erin Michos, who will share research about the dangers of sitting and what you can do about it. Hello, Erin, how does so much sitting affect health?

Michos: A large review of studies published in 2015 in the *Annals of Internal Medicine* found that even after adjusting for physical activity, sitting for long periods was associated with worse health outcomes including heart disease, Type 2 diabetes and cancer. Sedentary behavior can also increase your risk of dying, either from heart disease or other medical problems.

Reporter: Even fitness buffs can be sedentary, as you recently discovered?

Michos: I consider myself physically active. I run every morning for four or five miles, and I'd pat myself on the back for that. But then I got a step-tracking device and realized I wasn't moving much the rest of the day. I have a long commute, so I was spending two hours in my car. On days I'm not doing rounds, I'm doing research or teaching, so I might be sitting at my computer for eight hours. I was easily sitting more than 10 hours a day. Outside of my run, I was getting very few steps the rest of the day.

49

Reporter: Does all that sitting cancel out the benefits of your daily running?

Michos: Not entirely. More recent research shows that high levels of exercise can lessen some of the risk. Yet even for people with high levels of activity, there seems to be a threshold around 10 hours of sitting. Research shows that if you sit more than 10 hours, your cardiovascular risk really goes up.

Reporter: How have you changed your own habits?

Michos: I've made progress. I make an effort to get up and move around every hour. I try to find as many excuses as possible to walk throughout the day. I've also been having walking meetings. We'll do loops around the hospital and talk as we walk.

Reporter: What advice do you have to help others get out of their seats?

Michos: Even if you have to be sitting in front of the computer all day, you can break up the time. You don't have to replace sitting with time at the gym. There's benefit to light activity during the day. For every 20 minutes of sitting, try to stand for eight minutes and move around for two minutes. I recommend everybody track their steps, with a fitness tracker, your phone or a simple pedometer. We usually recommend a target of 10,000 steps a day.

Now you'll hear Part Two again. This is the end of Part Two. Now look at Part Three. You will hear a discussion among an instructor and two medical students. For questions 14—20, choose the most appropriate answer. Mark the corresponding letter on your answer sheet. You will hear the discussion twice.

Instructor: Today we are going to discuss cellulitis. Cellulitis is a bacterial infection of the dermis—the deep layer of skin—as well as the subcutaneous tissues, the fat and soft tissue layer that is under the skin.

Student 1: I learnt that some types of bacteria are naturally present on the skin and do not normally cause any harm.

Instructor: Yes. Bacteria from the streptococci and staphylococci groups are commonly found on the surface of the skin and cause no harm; however, if they enter the skin, they can cause infection. For the bacteria to access the deeper skin layers, they need a route in, which is usually through a break in the skin. A break in the skin can be caused by ulcers, burns, bites, grazes, cuts, and some skin conditions such as eczema, athlete's foot, or psoriasis. Some people even develop cellulitis without being able to identify a break in the skin.

Student 2: What are common symptoms for cellulitis?

Student 1: The affected area will become warm, tender, inflamed, swollen, red and painful.

Instructor: Right. Some people may develop blisters, skin dimpling, or spots. They might also experience a fever, chills, nausea, and shivering. Lymph glands may swell and become tender. If the cellulitis has affected the person's leg, the lymph glands in their groin may also be swollen or tender. So, what can we do to prevent cellulitis?

Student 1: If the skin is broken because of a cut, bite, or graze, it should be kept clean to reduce risk of infection.

Student 2: Reducing the likelihood of scratching and infecting the skin. The risk of the skin being damaged by scratching will be greatly reduced if fingernails are kept short and clean. Taking good care of the skin is also helpful. If the skin is dry, moisturizers should be used to prevent skin from cracking. However, individuals with greasy skin will not need to do this. Moisturizers will not help if the skin is already infected.

Instructor: Exactly! Because obesity may raise the risk of developing cellulitis, controlling weight should be paid attention to.

Student 1: After being infected, how to treat cellulitis?

Instructor: There is no way to treat cellulitis at home, and this condition needs to be treated by a doctor. If someone suspects they have cellulitis, they should call a doctor right away. Of course, there are something they can do. Drinking plenty of water, keeping the affected area raised, and taking painkillers are usually recommended by a doctor.

Student 2: How about using tea tree oil?

Instructor: Some people have suggested using tea tree oil, coconut oil, and garlic, because they may have antibacterial, antifungal, and other properties. However, there appears to be no evidence that they can treat cellulitis. Anyone with symptoms needs to seek medical help at once. Untreated, cellulitis can be life-threatening.

Now you'll hear Part Three again. This is the end of Part Three. Now look at Part Four. You will hear a speech on natural ways to adjust sleeping habits. Complete the notes. In each blank, write only one word. Write the answers on your answer sheet. You will hear the speech twice.

Male: Disturbed sleep is more than an inconvenience that leaves you dragging the next day: it can affect your emotional and physical health. It negatively affects your memory, concentration and mood, and it boosts your risk for depression, obesity, Type 2 diabetes, heart disease and high blood pressure.

Happily, there are easy, natural fixes that can improve your sleep. It's not always necessary to get a prescription for a sleep aid. There are natural ways to make adjustments to your sleeping habits.

No. 1 Drink up. Warm milk, chamomile tea and tart cherry juice are recommended for

51

patients with sleep trouble.

Warm milk has long been believed to be associated with chemicals that simulate the effects of tryptophan on the brain. This is a chemical building block for the substance serotonin, which is involved in the sleep-wake transition. Chamomile tea can also be helpful. It's believed to have flavonoids that may interact with benzodiazepine receptors in the brain that are also involved with the sleep-wake transition. Plus, chamomile tea doesn't have caffeine, unlike green tea or Earl Grey. Finally, tart cherry juice might support melatonin production and support a healthy sleep cycle.

No. 2 Exercise. It's known that moderate aerobic exercise boosts the amount of deep sleep you get. But you have to time it right. Aerobic exercise releases endorphins, chemicals that keep people awake. This is why you feel energized after a run. It can also raise core body temperature; this spike signals the body that it's time to get up and get going. If you're having trouble sleeping, try to avoid working out within two hours of bedtime.

No. 3 Use melatonin supplements. Melatonin is a hormone that is naturally released in the brain four hours before we feel a sense of sleepiness. It's triggered by the body's response to reducing light exposure, which should naturally happen at night.

These days, though, lights abound after it's dark outside—whether it's from your phone, laptop or TV. This exposure to unnatural light prevents melatonin release, which can make it hard to fall asleep. Luckily, melatonin is available in pill form at your local pharmacy as an over-the-counter supplement.

Just make sure that you consistently buy the same brand. Because melatonin supplements are unregulated by the FDA, the per-pill dosages and ingredients may differ from manufacturer to manufacturer. Stick with one brand, and don't buy it online from an unknown source.

No. 4 Keep cool. The ideal temperature for your thermostat is between 65 and 72 degrees. Women who are going through menopause and experiencing hot flashes should keep the room as cool as possible and wear cotton or breathable fabrics to bed.

No. 5 Go dark. It's known that the light from a smartphone interferes with sleep. But what about your bathroom light? If you have the urge to go at night, don't flick on the lights. The latest recommendation is to use a flashlight if you need to get up at night, because it offers less visual disruption. And remember: If you do wake up for a bathroom break, it might take up to 30 minutes to drift back off. This is completely normal.

Now you'll hear Part Four again. This is the end of Part Four. You now have five minutes to write your answers on the answer sheet. You have one more minute. This is the end of the listening test.

参考答案与试题评析

I Listening

Part One

1.【语段大意】医生通过对患者病史的了解,得知患者肺源性吸气胸痛(the pulmonary unit with chest pain on inspiration)、呼吸困难(dyspnea)、发汗(diaphoresis)。3 年前,患者对左肺原发性巨细胞肉瘤(primary giant cell sarcoma)进行了左肺叶切除术(a lobectomy of the left lung),随后进行放疗和化疗(radiation and chemotherapy)。医生提示吸烟对健康有害,每天吸 1/2 包香烟对 52 岁的人来说实在是太多了。戒烟确实是必要的。

【解题思路】E 可听到 smoking is bad for health, quitting smoking is really necessary 等关键信息。

2.【语段大意】医生正对患者子女讲述患者情况:患者在 ICU 处于多器官功能衰竭的末期(in the terminal stage of multisystem organ failure),有 20 年的慢性阻塞性肺疾病史(COPD),无意识、无法独自呼吸、动脉气血异常(Her ABGs are abnormal)。患者被诊断为难治性呼吸窘迫综合征(refractory ARDS)。医生建议永久性气管造口术(a permanent tracheostomy),家庭考虑继续或撤回生命支持。

【解题思路】C 可听到 in the terminal stage of multisystem organ failure, refractory ARDS, family consideration of continuing or withdrawing life support 等关键信息。

3.【语段大意】医生分析患者情况:入院检查(examination on admission)显示阳性墨菲征(a positive Murphy sign)的右上腹反跳痛(rebound tenderness in the RUQ),皮肤、指甲和结膜(skin, nails, and conjunctivae)是黄色的,白细胞计数(leukocyte count)是16 000,内镜逆行胰胆管造影术(ERCP)和腹部超声检查(ultrasound of the abdomen)提示胆囊(gallbladder)中可能有许多小结石(small stones),而且可能是在胆总管(the common bile duct)中。最终诊断是胆囊炎(cholecystitis)胆石症(cholelithiasis)。

【解题思路】B 可听到最后"Your diagnosis is cholecystitis with cholelithiasis."这一关键句。

4.【语段大意】医生分析患者情况:先前的(previous)钡灌肠(barium enema)显示了大肠(large bowel)的乙状结肠和直肠段(sigmoid and rectal segments)的一些不规则性(irregularities);粪便培养(stool samples for culture)、卵子(ova)和寄生虫(parasites)是阴性的(negative)。初步诊断(tentative diagnosis)是应激性肠综合征(irritable bowel syndrome)。医生提示遵循无乳糖低残留饮食(a lactose-free, low-residue diet),服用碘化钠(take Imodium)以减少肠道蠕动(reduce intestinal motility);建议做结肠镜检查(colonoscopy)。

【解题思路】D 可听到 large bowel, irritable bowel syndrome 等关键信息。

5.【语段大意】医生在为患者分析病因:患者从急诊室到住院部(admitted to the in-patient unit from the ER),右侧腹痛严重(severe right flank pain),对止痛药无反应(unresponsive to analgesics)。100 毫克 IV 哌替啶的给药(with administration of 100 mg of IV meperidine),疼痛并没有减少。患者有 3 个月的慢性泌尿系感染史(3-month history of chronic UTI)。问题可能是由六个月前开的低骨密度的钙补充剂(the calcium supplements for low bone density)引起的。

【解题思路】A　可听到 the calcium supplements，six months ago 等关键信息。

Part Two

【语篇大意】一名记者与心脏病专家埃林·米霍斯之间的对话，关于久坐的危险以及应对方法。

【解题思路】

6. B　对话开头就提到"体力劳动的工作占比不到 20％"，故答案为 B。

7. A　对话中提及"久坐会导致更坏的结果，包括心脏病(heart disease)、2 型糖尿病(Type 2 diabetes)和癌症(cancer)"，故答案为 A。

8. B　当记者问"健身爱好者也可以久坐不动吗"时，Michos 说"我认为自己热衷于锻炼身体。我每天早上跑步四到五英里，对此我要给自己点赞。但后来我用了一个计步的跟踪装置，并意识到我在一天中剩下的时间里都没有移动……"，题干中"leads a completely healthy lifestyle"不对，所以答案为 B。

9. C　原文"研究表明，如果你坐超过 10 小时，你的心血管风险(cardiovascular risk)确实上升"，没有提心脏病风险，所以选 C。

10. B　原文"最近的研究表明，高水平的运动可以减少一些风险"，题干中"have no cardiovascular risk"没有风险不对，因此选 B。

11. A　Michos 说"我也参加过散步会议。我们绕着医院，边走边说话"，所以选 A。

12. A　Michos 说"即使你必须整天坐在电脑前，你也可以合理拆分时间"，所以选 A。

13. B　Michos 说"我们通常推荐每天 10 000 步的目标"，而非 11 000 步，故选 B。

Part Three

【语篇大意】老师与两位学生在讨论蜂窝组织炎(cellulitis)的引发、症状、预防和治疗。

【解题思路】

14. A　对话开头提及"蜂窝组织炎是一种细菌感染真皮——深层皮肤、皮下组织、脂肪组织层下的皮肤"，故 A 为答案。关键信息：Cellulitis is a bacterial infection of the dermis—the deep layer of skin—as well as the subcutaneous tissues，the fat and soft tissue layer that is under the skin.

15. C　对话中提到"皮肤破裂可能是由溃疡、烧伤、咬伤、擦伤、伤口和一些皮肤疾病如湿疹、脚癣或银屑病引起的"，没有 swelling(肿胀)，故答案为 C。关键信息：A break in the skin can be caused by ulcers，burns，bites，grazes，cuts，and some skin conditions such as eczema，athlete's foot，or psoriasis.

16. B　对话中提到"蜂窝组织炎的常见症状：受影响的区域会发热、组织变软、发炎、肿胀、红肿和疼痛。有些人可能会出现水疱、皮肤凹陷或斑点。他们也可能经历发烧、寒战、恶心和颤抖。淋巴结可能肿胀并变得柔软。"，没有 inflammation of lymph glands 淋巴结发炎，所以答案应该选 B。关键信息：The affected area will become warm，tender，inflamed，swollen，red and painful. Some people may develop blisters，skin dimpling，or spots. They might also experience a fever，chills，nausea，and shivering. Lymph glands may

swell and become tender.

17. B　对话中提到"如果皮肤因割伤、咬伤或擦伤而破裂,应保持清洁,以减少感染的风险。减少搔痒和感染皮肤的可能性。如果指甲保持短而干净,皮肤划伤的风险会大大降低。如果皮肤干燥,应使用保湿剂来预防皮肤开裂。然而,油腻皮肤的人不需要这样做。如果皮肤已经被感染,保湿剂将无济于事。由于肥胖可能会增加蜂窝组织炎的风险,应重视体重控制。"avoid using of moisturizers(使用保湿霜)是有前提条件的,故答案为B。关键信息:If the skin is broken because of a cut, bite, or graze, it should be kept clean to reduce risk of infection. Reducing the likelihood of scratching and infecting the skin. The risk of the skin being damaged by scratching will be greatly reduced if fingernails are kept short and clean. Taking good care of the skin is also helpful. If the skin is dry, moisturizers should be used to prevent skin from cracking. However, individuals with greasy skin will not need to do this. Moisturizers will not help if the skin is already infected. Because obesity may raise the risk of developing cellulitis, controlling weight should be paid attention to.

18. C　对话中提到"家里没有办法治疗蜂窝组织炎,这种情况需要去看医生",显然C正确。关键信息:There is no way to treat cellulitis at home, and this condition needs to be treated by a doctor.

19. A　对话中提到"有些人建议使用茶树油、椰子油和大蒜,因为它们可能具有抗菌、抗真菌和其他特性",故答案为A。关键信息:Some people have suggested using tea tree oil, coconut oil, and garlic, because they may have antibacterial, antifungal, and other properties.

20. B　对话最后提到"然而,似乎没有证据表明他们可以治疗蜂窝组织炎。任何有症状的人都需要立即寻求医疗帮助。未经治疗,蜂窝组织炎可能危及生命",故答案为B。关键信息:However, there appears to be no evidence that they can treat cellulitis. Anyone with symptoms needs to seek medical help at once. Untreated, cellulitis can be life-threatening.

Part Four

【语篇大意】一个关于调整睡眠习惯方法的演讲。

【解题思路】

21. milk　此处为演讲中提到的第一个调整睡眠习惯的方法,即喝一杯温牛奶、洋甘菊茶或酸樱桃汁。所以此处应填 milk。

22. aerobic　此处为演讲中提到的第二个调整睡眠习惯的方法,即锻炼。众所周知,适度的有氧运动能增加你的深度睡眠。所以此处应填 aerobic。

23. hormone　此处为演讲中提到的第三个调整睡眠习惯的方法,即使用褪黑激素补充剂。褪黑激素是一种荷尔蒙,在我们感觉昏昏欲睡之前四小时内自然释放。所以此处应填 hormone。

24. menopause　此处为演讲中提到的第四个调整睡眠习惯的方法,即保持凉爽。经历更年期和潮热的妇女应尽量保持房间的凉爽。故此处应填 menopause。

25. disruption　此处为演讲中提到的第五个调整睡眠习惯的方法,即使周围变暗。如果你需要在晚上起床，最好使用手电筒，因为手电筒的视觉干扰比电灯小。故此处应填 disruption。

Ⅱ Reading

Part One

【文章大意】文章描述了美国蛋类生产商玫瑰农场，因环境卫生不合格和员工的不规范操作而导致沙门氏菌爆发的来龙去脉，并在文章结尾指出了沙门氏菌的传染途径和感染后的各种不良后果。

【解题思路】从列表 A 到 F 中选择每个段落的最合适的副标题。

26．C　根据第一段第一句、第三句和第四句可以断定选 C。本段描述了第一起沙门氏菌感染病例以及疾病爆发后追查到其中 35 人致病原因为食用存在鼠患的同一农场蛋产品。

27．B　根据第二段第二句至最后一句，都是直接引述该蛋产品生产商的道歉和承诺。

28．A　根据第三段第二句至最后一句，都是描述检查人员在该农场发现的各类卫生状况和雇员不规范的生产操作行为。

29．E　根据第四段第一句"The 'unsanitary conditions and poor employee practices' created an environment that allowed for pathogens that could cause egg contamination to thrive throughout the facility, the report says."为中心句，其余部分是人们对该问题的控诉，均为支撑细节。

30．D　第五段第一句就是说明沙门氏菌的来源；第二句至最后一句在描述健康人群感染沙门氏菌表现的症状以及沙门氏菌对幼儿和年老人群可能造成的严重后果。

31．A　定位第一段第一句"... 'unacceptable rodent activity' had been going on at the facility for months, before the first of the salmonella-related illnesses occurred but the facility's management did not take appropriate actions and unsanitary practices continued."。

32．C　定位第二段倒数第二句"When we fall short of expectations, we're disappointed in ourselves and we strive to correct any problems and institute safeguards that ensure those problems won't occur again."。

33．D　定位第三段第三句"A few carcasses were found lying in and outside the houses."。

34．F　定位第四段倒数第二句"Eggs produced at the farm are distributed to retail stores and restaurants in Colorado, Florida, New Jersey, New York, Pennsylvania, Virginia, West Virginia and the Carolinas."。

35．B　定位第五段第一句"Salmonella can come from contaminated animal products such as beef, poultry, milk and eggs, as well as fruits and vegetables."。

Part Two

【文章大意】文章主要介绍了阿尔茨海默氏症的定义、病因、症状以及缓解病情的可行手段。

【解题思路】

36．A　根据第六段第一句"Alzheimer's disease is the most common cause of dementia, which is a collective term for symptoms including problems with language and thinking, and commonly memory loss. "得知 A 选项正确。

37. C 文章第七段"导致阿尔茨海默氏症的原因是什么?"紧接着第八段开头给出了概述"This is still poorly understood. "因此选 C。

38. D 根据第八段第三句"However there are several factors which increase the risk, with age being the biggest, one sufferer in 20 is less risk than that under the age of 65 ... "得知年龄是增加阿尔茨海默氏症患病风险的最大因素,年龄越大,患病风险越高。故 A、C 选项错误。同时,第九段提到"There are twice as many women with Alzheimer's over the age 65 as men ... "65 岁以上患阿尔茨海默氏的女性是男性的两倍,可知女性患病几率更大,B 选项错误。

39. B 根据第九段第一句"Lifestyle factors including smoking, obesity and diet are another major factor in increasing risk",提到了增加阿尔茨海默氏症患病风险的另一主要因素包括吸烟、肥胖和饮食在内的生活方式。得知 B 选项正确。

40. B 根据第十一段第一句"Depression can be a very early sign which may occur before any physical hallmarks in the brain. "得知是 before ,不是 after,B 为正确答案。

41. D 根据文章第十三段第一句话"There is no cure for the disease, though this is a major research area along with developing tests for earlier diagnosis. "(虽然这是一个主要的研究领域,同时也在开发早期诊断的测试,但是这种疾病还没有治愈的方法。)因此选 D。

42. B 最后一段第三句话总述了药物治疗仅可以缓解症状"There are drug treatments which can temporarily improve some symptoms. "第四、五句话分述了早期阶段和后期阶段分别可以使用哪些药物来缓解哪些症状。因此 B 选项正确,而其他三个选项均有错误。

Part Three

【文章大意】文章阐述了结直肠癌及化疗的副作用,化学佐剂西洋参可以降低化疗的毒性,研究数据表明西洋参浆果有可能提高 5-FU 的肿瘤杀伤作用。

【解题思路】

43. B 根据第一段第一句"Colorectal cancer is one of the most common malignancies and ranks as the second greatest cause of cancer death in both men and women worldwide. "结直肠癌是第二大癌症死亡原因,因此题目错误。

44. A 根据第二段第五句"American ginseng has been reported to have stress-relieving qualities, anti-aging effects and digestion-aiding effects. "(据报道,西洋参具有缓解压力的品质,抗衰老的功效和助消化作用。)题目正确。

45. A 根据第三段第四句"The 5-Fluorouracil (5-FU) is one of the most widely used chemotherapeutic agents in first-line therapy for colorectal cancer, and an overall survival benefit after fluorouracil-based chemotherapy has been firmly established. "[5-氟尿嘧啶(5-FU)是目前在大肠癌一线治疗中应用最广泛的化疗药物之一,氟脲基化疗后的整体生存效果已被肯定。]题目正确。

46. C 题目意思是"这些化合物的浓度随遗传、季节、地理分布、植物生长、生产和提取过程的不同而有显著差异"。此信息在文中没有给出,故选 C。

47. C 题目意思是"目前尚不清楚在化疗时使用西洋参浆果提取物是否会影响化疗药物的疗效"。此信息在文中并未涉及,故选 C。

48. B 根据第四段最后一句话"The successful treatment regimens for cancer include combination chemotherapy, which is often more effective than single chemotherapy because of additive or synergistic effects."(癌症的成功治疗方案包括联合化疗,由于附加或协同作用,联合化疗通常比单一化疗更有效。)关键词 more,对比可知题目错误。

49. B 根据第五段第二句"Our data suggest that AGBE has the potential to heighten the tumoricidal effects of 5-FU and that 5-FU-induced antiproliferation of human colorectal cancer cells can be strengthened by combination with AGBE."(我们的数据表明,AGBE 有可能提高 5-FU 的肿瘤杀伤作用,而 5-FU 诱导的人类结直肠癌细胞的抗增殖能力可以通过与 AGBE 结合得到加强。)关键词 can be 可知,题目错误。

50. A 根据第五段最后一句话"The mechanism may include the enhancement of AGBE on the Sand G2/M phases arrest and the expression level of cyclin A, but not the induction of cell apoptosis."(这一机制可能包括增强沙 G2/M 期 AGBE 抑制和 cyclin A 的表达水平,而不是诱导细胞凋亡。)题目正确。

Part Four

【文章大意】文章用研究例证的方式阐述了乐观对身体健康的影响:与寿命有关;在疾病和疾病的康复中的积极作用(乳腺癌、动脉粥样硬化);影响人的免疫系统;对免疫受损的人的影响。

【解题思路】

51. D 第一段第一句是段落主题句,指出乐观与寿命有关。并用两个研究例证来佐证。第一个是 2000 年 Maruta, Colligan, Malinchoc 和 Offord 的研究;第二个是 20 世纪 60 年代中期的研究,将病人分为乐观、混合或悲观。其中对于乐观的研究运用了明尼苏达州的人格量表,并得出了 51 题的发现:一个人的乐观程度分数每增加 10 分,早逝的风险就会减少 19%。有助于正确选题的重要词句包括 Maruta, Colligan, Malinchoc, and Offord (2000) examined/With a large longitudinal sample collected in the mid-1960s, the researchers categorized/ using parts of the Minnesota Multiphasic Personality Inventory.

52. A 第三段第一句是段落主题句,指出乐观态度也在疾病和疾病的康复中起重要作用。52 题开始就用研究例证来支持这一论点。第四段开头"这些研究发现"和文中的"乳腺癌"提示 52 题选择多项研究调查了乐观在癌症治疗中的作用。有助于正确选题的重要词句包括 recovery from illness and disease/These studies have found that/ breast cancer。

53. E 第四段提到了乐观在乳腺癌治疗中的积极作用;社交活动的作用;睡眠质量;53 题预防慢性疾病发展的作用(例证:动脉粥样硬化)。有助于正确选题的重要词句包括 breast cancer/social activities/sleep quality/atherosclerosis(动脉粥样硬化)

54. C 第五段第一句话是段落主题句,指出乐观也会影响人的免疫系统。分别用老人接种流感疫苗和法学院学生的性格乐观来例证。段落最后指出这项研究发现乐观预示了细胞介导的免疫能力,这是免疫系统对感染因子反应的重要组成部分。此外,负面影响也不能预测免疫功能的变化。引出最后一句 54 题这就意味着乐观确实在免疫系统中的独特价值。有助于正确选题的重要词句包括 Optimism can have an effect on a person's immune

system，as well/ This study found that optimism predicted superior cell-mediated immunity/Furthermore，negative affect did not predict changes in immune function/ What this means is that/ unique value。

55. B 最后一段是总结段落,本句话55题"上述研究有一个共同的主题:乐观对一个人的身体健康有深远的影响"也是对全篇例证的一个总结。有助于正确选题的重要词句包括 boost a person's immune system/ protect against harmful behaviors /prevent chronic disease/and help people cope following troubling news/ predict a longer life。

Part Five

【文章大意】文章介绍了肾脏移植的一些情况,肾胰腺移植的例子以及影响移植的一些因素。

【解题思路】

56. C typically 是副词,典型地,这个地方要用副词修饰动词 classified,atypically 词意表达不准确。

57. B transplanted,这句话表达的意思是:有时候,肾脏可以跟胰腺一起移植。

58. A 本句"Only a few living donor pancreas transplants have been done"表达只有少数的人胰腺移植成功。用 a few 来修饰可数名词人,表示有一些,但是 few 表示几乎没有人,与文章的意思相悖。

59. D 根据"but even 75-year-old recipients gain an average of four more years of life",说明前面应该是意为年轻的会有更好的结果,故选 D,younger 较年轻的,而 young 是年轻人,这里表达比六七十岁更年轻的,不只是年轻人。

60. C 这里想表达"除了……之外还有……",故选 C,away from, far from 是表达远离……; suffer from 是遭受某种疾病。

61. A 文中"For example, different socio-demographic groups express different interest and complete pre-transplant _____ at different rates."意思为:"比如不同的社会层次有不同的兴趣,也以不同的速度来完成移植前的检查。"pre-transplant 是移植前的,选项中 work out 解决,算出,workout 为锻炼、练习,work up 建立发展,只有 A 选项 workup 意为诊断检查,故选 A。

62. B "Previous efforts to create fair transplantation policies have focused on patients currently on the transplantation waiting list."此处意为:"以前为制定公平的移植政策所做的努力集中在目前在移植等待名单的病人身上。"选 B 符合语义。

63. B 此处译为:"在接受肾移植的患者中,达到耐受度仍然是一个非常理想的目标。"仍然用 remain,注意主谓一致,故选 B。

64. D 首先是从时态上排除,前面有 have,故此处为完成时态,排除 B,C。此处表达:对自发的肾移植受者的机械性研究发现了 B 或调节 T 细胞的潜在作用,故选 D uncovered,揭露,发现。

65. A "... distinct protocols at three major transplant centers have _____ successful withdrawal of immunosuppression ..."此句句意为:"在三个主要的移植中心有不同的协议导致了活体供肾移植受者的免疫抑制成功地退出。"lead to 意为导致,选其他选项句子意思均不符合常理或逻辑。

III Writing

66.【范文】

In recent years, the relationship between doctors and patients has come under heated discussion among general public. With the tensions increase, it is imperative to find out some ways to ease the tense relations. In my stance, mutual understanding and health care improvement are the two most important aspects that should be taken to solve the problem.

First, to effectively ease the current tensions of doctor-patient relationship, understanding between doctors and patients and their families should be enhanced. To be specific, doctors should fulfill their obligations to inform the patients about the details of their condition, including the patients' diagnosis and treatment options. In the meantime, they should offer the most appropriate treatment for the patients, and give advice from a professional point of view. Conversely, patients should actively cooperate with the doctors with complete trust.

In addition, the health care system should be improved step by step. Another possible cause for the tense of doctor-patient lies in the inadequate health care system. The way doctors receive their salary and bonus, the drug regulation, and the percentage of medical expenses and medical insurance paid by patients themselves are underlying reasons for the worsening relationship between doctors and patients. From this perspective, to ease the conflicts, the government should try to optimize the health care system by mild revolution of the above specific aspects.

All in all, it is high time that doctors, patients and the government should make joint effort to deal with the poor relationship. Only in this way can we create a harmonious doctor-patient relationship. (255 words)

【审题】

写作部分要求围绕"医患关系"进行写作。题目陈述了近年来,医患关系日趋紧张和复杂,医患纠纷愈演愈烈,医疗活动和医院的正常秩序受到严重影响这一社会现象,要求就如何处理好医患关系提出一些建议。文章应属说明文,写作中的一个重点是能就造成医患关系恶化的原因给出可行性建议,难点是如何正确写出一些涉及医疗卫生领域话题的英语表达,如"医护人员、医疗体系、医疗费用、药品监管"等。

【范文评析】

文章首先根据题目要求,指出解决医患关系迫在眉睫,并明确提出两点建议。第二段第一句总领全段,随后从医生和患者自身该如何做给出具体建议。第三段第一句总领全段,随后提出政府可从三方面着手改革。

文章观点明确,两个主题句有效支持全文主旨句,阐述合理,展开充分;语言表达准确,特别是使用了"to some extent""step by step""possible cause""mildly"等模糊限制语,精准地表达了作者的观点。

医护英语水平考试(三级)

模拟训练(六)

听力文本

This is METS-3 listening test. There are four parts in the test, Part One, Two, Three, and Four. You will hear each part twice. We will now stop for a moment before we start the test. Please ask any questions now because you must not speak during the test. Now, look at the instructions for Part One.

You will hear five extracts from conversations taking place in different clinical departments. Choose which case each doctor is discussing from the list A—F. Use each letter A—F only once. There is one extra letter which you do not need to use. Mark the corresponding letter on your answer sheet. You will hear each extract twice. Now we are ready to start.

Extract 1

I have read your report. You have had chronic glomerulonephritis since age 7. And you have been managed at home with CAPD for the last 16 months as waiting a kidney transplant. I advise you to go immediately to the ER when you feel chest pain, shortness of breath, and oliguria.

Extract 2

I advise a surgical referral. You are diagnosed with bilateral direct inguinal hernias and I suggest that you not delay surgery, though you are not at high risk for a strangulated hernia. About your question that whether you can also be sterilized at the same time, you can be scheduled for bilateral inguinal herniorrhaphy and elective vasectomy.

Extract 3

I don't recommend hormone therapy, because I think you are at too much risk for excessive bleeding with the abnormal cells on your cervix. Don't forget you just spent 3 months under the care of gynecologist for treatment of postmenopausal bleeding and cervical dysplasia. Not to mention the several vaginal examinations with Pap smears, a uterine ultrasound, colposcopy with endocervical biopsies, and a D&C with cone biopsy.

Extract 4

You have an uneventful pregnancy with good health, moderate weight gain, good fetal heart sounds, and no signs or symptoms of pregnancy-induced hypertension. X-ray pelvimetry reveals CPD with the fetus in right occiput posterior position. Changes in fetal heart rate indicate fetal distress. You will be transported to the OR for emergency C-section under spinal anesthesia.

Extract 5

You should know that severe pancreatitis has a mortality rate near 50%. It's lucky that you have survived heart surgery, but to now we really have to worry about multisystem organ failure. What's worse, you have severe stabbing midepigastric pain that radiates to your back, nausea, vomiting, abdominal distention and rigidity, and jaundice.

Now you'll hear Part One again. This is the end of Part One. Now look at Part Two.
You will hear a conversation between a reporter and a transplantation expert. For each of the following statements, decide whether it is True (A) or False (B). If there is not enough information to answer True (A) or False (B), choose Not Given (C). Mark the corresponding letter on your answer sheet. You will hear the recording twice.

Reporter: I am Cecilia Austin. It is reported that nearly 124, 000 men, women and children are awaiting organ transplants in the United States. Every 10 minutes, another name is added to the national organ transplant waiting list. Twenty-one people die each day from lack of a transplant.

A living donor can eliminate the need for a recipient to be added to the national waiting list. I am interviewing Andrew MacGregor Cameron, a Johns Hopkins transplantation expert. He will answer frequently asked questions about live organ donation. Dr. Cameron, who can become a living donor?

Cameron: Living donors must be at least 18 years old, in good physical and mental health, and must have a body mass index that is less than 35. Living donors can be relatives, friends, neighbors, in-laws or altruistic strangers.

Reporter: Altruistic strangers?

Cameron: Yes, individuals who wish to donate to an unknown recipient purely out of selfless motives.

Reporter: What can I donate?

Cameron: As a living donor, you can donate one of your kidneys and part of your liver.

Reporter: What are the risks and recovery for a living organ donor?

Cameron: Just like with any other major surgery, there are risks and a period of critical recovery time for transplantation surgery. For kidney donors, the remaining kidney will enlarge slightly because it has to do the work of two healthy kidneys. For liver donors, the liver regenerates and regains full function. The recovery time after surgery is typically six to eight weeks. Living donation does not change life expectancy. Most donors go on to live healthy lives after recovering from the surgery. Specific donor-related risks should be discussed with your transplant team.

Reporter: Can I donate my organs if I have a medical condition?

Cameron: Possibly. Most people can donate, but there are a few exclusions, such as HIV, active cancer and systemic infection. Your doctors will evaluate your medical condition and the condition of your organs to determine if you are qualified to be a living organ donor.

Reporter: Who pays for the cost of an organ donation?

Cameron: In most cases, the transplant recipient's private health insurance, Medicare or Medicaid will pay for the donor's initial evaluation, surgery and postoperative care.

Reporter: Can non-US citizens donate organs?

Cameron: Yes. Non-US citizens can receive and donate organs in the United States.

Reporter: Can I sell my organs?

Cameron: All live kidney and liver donations must be a completely voluntary decision. Donors should be free from any pressure or guilt associated with the donation, and they cannot be paid for their donation. In 1984, Congress passed the National Organ Transplant Act, which makes it illegal to buy or sell organs.

Reporter: How can I become a donor?

Cameron: If you are interested in donating a kidney to someone in need, please call 410 - 614 - 9345 or register online. If you are interested in donating a liver to someone in need, please call 410 - 614 - 2989.

Now you'll hear Part Two again. This is the end of Part Two. Now look at Part Three. You will hear a discussion among an instructor and two medical students. For questions 14—20, choose the best appropriate answer. Mark the corresponding letter on your answer sheet. You will hear the discussion twice.

Instructor: Today we are going to discuss breast cancer. It is the most common cancer in women worldwide, with nearly 1.7 million new cases diagnosed in 2012. This represents about 12% of all new cancer cases and 25% of all cancers in women. It is the fifth most common cause of death from cancer in women. Who would like to start?

Student 1: Breast cancer risk doubles each decade until menopause, after which the increase slows. However, breast cancer is more common after menopause.

Student 2: Survival rates for breast cancer vary worldwide, but in general the rates have improved. This is because breast cancer is diagnosed at an earlier and localised stage in nations where populations have access to medical care, and progressive improvement in treatment strategies.

Instructor: Yes. In many countries with advanced medical care, the five-year survival rate of early stage breast cancers is 80—90 percent, falling to 24 percent for breast cancers diagnosed at a more advanced stage. Most breast cancer subtypes are hormone-related. The natural history of the disease differs between those diagnosed before and after the menopause, which may be due to different kinds of tumour and possibly different effects of nutritional factors on hormones depending on menopausal status.

Student 1: What are the risk factors for breast cancer?

Instructor: Life events are important risk factors for breast cancer including early menarche, late natural menopause, not bearing children and first pregnancy over the age of 30, as they all increase lifetime exposure to oestrogen and progesterone and the risk of breast cancer.

Student 2: So the reverse also applies that late menarche, early menopause, bearing children and pregnancy before the age of 30 all reduce the risk of breast cancer.

Instructor: You are right. In addition, ionising radiation exposure from medical treatment such as X-rays, particularly during puberty, increases the risk of breast cancer, even at low doses.

Student 1: Does hormone therapy have any correlation with breast cancer?

Instructor: The answer is yes. Hormone therapy containing oestrogen with or without progesterone increases risk of breast cancer and the risk is greater with combined oestrogen plus progesterone preparations. Plus, oral contraceptives containing both oestrogen and progesterone also cause a small increased risk of breast cancer in young women, among current and recent users only.

Student 2: How about the prevalance of breast caner worldwide?

Instructor: In general, the highest incidence of breast cancer was in Northern America and Oceania, and the lowest incidence was in Asia and Africa. This is the table showing the countries with the top 20 highest incidence of breast cancer in 2012. You can see that Belgium had the highest rate of breast cancer, followed by Denmark and the Netherlands. Slightly more cases of breast cancer, that is, 53%, were diagnosed in less developed countries.

Now you'll hear Part Three again. This is the end of Part Three. Now look at Part Four. You will hear a speech on helpful strategies after receiving a dementia diagnosis. Complete the notes. In each blank, write only one word. Write the answers on your answer sheet. You will hear the speech twice.

Male: When you or a loved one first receives a dementia diagnosis, you may feel a range of contradictory emotions, sometimes simultaneously. Many people undergo a period of profound grief, with feelings of shock, denial and deep sadness. The prospect of facing this significant life change can make you feel demoralized, embarrassed or angry. You may even want to keep the diagnosis secret from friends or other family members.

On the other hand, you may feel a sense of relief. Finally, your suspicions have been validated, and you and your loved ones can seek out more support and therapeutic interventions.

Even after you've accepted the diagnosis, your emotions can vary depending on the situation—the stage of the illness, your financial and social resources, and so on. Your best move—for you and your loved one—is to be educated and prepared, and here some strategies can help.

Allow yourself time to adjust. The shock of the diagnosis can be paralyzing. Be gentle and compassionate with yourself; allow yourself to move through the mourning process. Try to feel all the feelings, rather than deny them, and be up-front with your family and friends about your diagnosis. You'll likely move into problem-solving mode faster.

Set up routines and expectations. People with dementia don't always believe they need help, so power struggles can ensue over daily tasks, warns Johnston. Clearly defined routines and predictable schedules for tasks such as cleaning and eating may help avoid some conflicts and help you both feel more settled. Orderly, peaceful environments also create calm.

Find an experienced dementia care counselor for both of you. One of Johnston's studies found that when caregivers and people with dementia sought treatment for depression, they gained greater access to care, services and support. Caregivers should have someone to talk to regularly, who can provide support, educate them about the illness and coach them on how to cope as it progresses.

Give each other space. As the disease progresses, rapidly swinging moods and angry, negative outbursts can take a great toll on caregivers. Plus, more than 90 percent of people with dementia develop behavioral symptoms or psychiatric problems at some point during their illness. It's perfectly OK to calmly say, "I need to have some privacy," and leave the room to have a moment of peace, to allow both of you to calm down.

Pace yourself. Caregivers may have trouble sleeping due to worry over their loved one's needs, yet still not have anyone to relieve them the next day when they're exhausted. The weight of all of these concerns can cause even the most resolute caregivers to experience stress, resentment and even depression. Rest when you can, and prioritize. Keep the day structured and predictable as much as possible, the environment uncluttered and activities simple.

Make time for daily exercise. A daily walk in a park or just around the block can be an effective antidepressant and antianxiety remedy for both of you. If needed, keep a sturdy transport wheelchair stowed in the trunk to broaden your options for walks together while running errands.

Now you'll hear Part Four again. This is the end of Part Four. You now have five minutes to write your answers on the answer sheet. You have one more minute. This is the end of the listening test.

参考答案与试题评析

Ⅰ Listening

Part One

1.【语段大意】医生通过患者的报告了解到,患者从 7 岁起就患有慢性肾小球肾炎(chronic glomerulonephritis)。在过去的 16 个月里,一直在家中接受(持续性非卧床式)腹膜透析[CAPD(Continuous Ambulatory Peritoneal Dialysis)]的治疗,等待肾脏移植。医生建议,当患者感到胸痛、气短和少尿时,应立即去看急诊。

【解题思路】F 可听到 chronic glomerulonephritis, waiting a kidney transplant 等关键信息。

2.【语段大意】患者被诊断为双侧腹股沟直疝,医生建议立即手术。关于患者提到是否可以同时进行绝育手术的问题,医生说可以安排双侧腹股沟疝修补术和择期输精管切除术。

【解题思路】C 可听到"I suggest that you not delay surgery"这一关键信息。

3.【语段大意】医生不建议患者接收激素治疗,因为患者宫颈有异常细胞并有过度出血的风险。

【解题思路】B 听力开始部分提到"I don't recommend hormone therapy"这一关键信息。

4.【语段大意】医生陈述这位孕妇身体健康,体重增加适度,胎儿心音良好,没有妊娠高血压的迹象或症状。但骨盆 X 线测量显示 CPD 与胎儿在右后枕位,胎儿心率的变化表明胎儿窘迫,医生认为患者需要剖宫产。

【解题思路】D 可听到 pregnancy, fetus 等关键词。

5.【语段大意】医生认为患者心脏手术很成功,但患者罹患重症胰腺炎,这种疾病的死亡率接近 50%,医生担心患者出现多系统器官衰竭。

【解题思路】E 听力开头部分可听到"You should know that severe pancreatitis has a mortality rate near 50%."这一关键句。

Part Two

【语篇大意】一位记者对一位移植专家关于器官移植的采访。

【解题思路】

6. A　记者提到每天有 21 人因未进行(器官)移植而死亡,故答案为 A。

7. B　专家提到,活体捐献者必须年满 18 岁,身心健康,体重指数必须小于 35。故答案为 B。

8. A　专家提到,活体捐献者可捐出一个肾脏和一部分肝脏。所以答案为 A。

9. C　专家提到肾脏捐献者的剩余肾脏会稍微增大,未提及手术后的恢复事项,所以 C 正确。

10. A　专家提到,活体捐赠不会影响寿命,因此选 A。

11. B　专家提到除艾滋病、癌症和全身性感染患者不能捐赠器官外,大部分人即使有健康问题也可以捐赠器官。所以选 B。

12. C　专家提到,在大多数情况下,移植接受者的私人健康保险、医疗保险或医疗补助将用于支付捐赠者的初步评估、手术和术后护理费用,但并未提及捐赠者是否会得到一笔术后护理费,所以选 C。

13. A　专家提到,1984 年,国会通过了"国家器官移植法案",规定买卖器官是非法的,故 A 正确。

Part Three

【语篇大意】两位医学生与老师讨论乳腺癌的相关问题。

【解题思路】

14. B　对话中提到,乳腺癌是妇女最常见的癌症,2012 年诊断出近 170 万例新病例,故答案为 B。

15. A　对话中提到,乳腺癌风险每十年增加一倍,直至绝经期,故答案为 A。

16. A　对话中提到,全世界乳腺癌的存活率各不相同,但总的说来,生存率有所提高。所以答案应该选 A。关键信息:Survival rates for breast cancer vary worldwide, but in general rates have improved.

17. C　对话中提到,在许多拥有先进医疗服务的国家,早期乳腺癌的 5 年生存率为 80%—90%,在晚期(advanced stage)被诊断为乳腺癌的生存率降至 24%,故答案为 C。关键信息:In many countries with advanced medical care, the five-year survival rate of early stage breast cancers is 80—90 percent, falling to 24 percent for breast cancers diagnosed at a more advanced stage.

18. C　对话中提到,月经初潮早、自然更年晚、不生育、30 岁以上第一次怀孕都增加了终生接触雌激素和黄体酮,以及患乳腺癌的风险。显然 C 正确。

关键信息:Life events are important risk factors for breast cancer including early menarche, late natural menopause, not bearing children and first pregnancy over the age of 30, as they all increase lifetime exposure to oestrogen and progesterone and the risk of breast cancer.

19. B　对话中提到含有雌激素的激素治疗,不管有没有黄体酮,都会增加乳腺癌的风险,雌激素加黄体酮联合制剂的风险更大。A 为雄激素,C 为睾丸素,故答案为 B。关键信息:Hormone therapy containing oestrogen with or without progesterone increases risk of breast cancer and the risk is greater with combined oestrogen plus progesterone preparations.

20. B　对话中提到,老师展示了 2012 年乳腺癌发病率最高的 20 个国家,并明确指出,比利时的乳腺癌发病率最高,其次是丹麦和荷兰。故答案为 B。关键信息:This is the table showing the countries with the top 20 highest incidence of breast cancer in 2012. You can see that Belgium had the highest rate of breast cancer, followed by Denmark and the Netherlands.

Part Four

【语篇大意】关于如何应对自己或家人痴呆诊断的一段讲座。

【解题思路】

21. compassionate　此处为讲座中提到的第一个策略,即给自己一些调整的时间,要对自己温柔体恤,允许自己经历这个悲伤的过程。所以此处应填 compassionate。

22. counselor　讲座中提到,可以找一位有经验的痴呆症护理顾问,所以此处应填 counselor。

23. psychiatric　讲座中提到,超过 90% 的痴呆症患者在患病期间会出现行为症状或精神问题。所以此处应填 psychiatric。

24. predictable　讲座中提到,应尽量保持一天的有序性和可预见性,保持环境整洁,活动简单。所以此处应填 predictable。

25. antidepressant　讲座最后提到,应保持每天运动,每天在公园或街区附近散步可有效抵御抑郁和焦虑。故此处应填 antidepressant。

II　Reading

Part One

【文章大意】文章论述了手机使用和健康之间的关系,并给出了一些使用手机的建议。

【解题思路】

26. C　第一段第三句和第四句就手机是否对身体产生危害提出两种研究结论:一类研究认为只有频繁使用者具有较大的罹患脑瘤的风险,而另一类研究表明使用手机和癌症之间并无联系。

27. F　第二段第三和第四句描述了两方面因素对当前研究的影响,一是使用手机与癌症形成之间的时间问题,二是来自手机制造商或个人利益可能对研究结论造成的影响。

28. B　第三段第二句"Mobile phone antennas are similar to microwave ovens.",第四句"Microwave ovens have radio wave frequencies that are high enough to cook food, and they are also known to be dangerous to human tissues like those in the brain.",以及第五句 "The concern is that the lower-frequency radio waves that mobile phones rely on may also be dangerous."表明,手机天线和微波炉相似,而众所周知,微波炉对身体组织会产生危害,所以,手机依赖的低频无线电波可能是危险的。

29. A　第四段第二、第三和第四句都是研究者提出的建议。

30. E　第五段第一句就指出手机使用者目前对手机的危害还没有足够的警觉;第四句以烟草为例,证明现在人们对手机的危害的认知就好比以前对烟草和肺癌之间的关联性的认知;第五、第六句描述了 2016 年的研究结果:大鼠脑瘤患病率的上升与手机发射的无线电频率有关。

31. C　定位第一段第三句"Some research suggests that heavy users of mobile phones are at a greater risk of developing cancerous brain tumors."。

32. D　定位第二段最后一句"Another concern about these studies is that many have been funded by the mobile phone industry or those who benefit from it."。

33. A　定位第三段第四句"The concern is that the lower-frequency radio waves that mobile phones rely on may also be dangerous."。

34. B　定位第四段第三句"They also say that many cordless phones can emit dangerous levels of Electromagnetic Radiation even when they are not in use."。

35. F　定位第五段最后一句"As a result, many experts now recommend texting or using head sets or speaker phones instead of holding a mobile phone to the ear."。

Part Two

【文章大意】文章讲述了Gough对于自己的妻子因为乳腺癌筛查出现错误,而错失最佳的治疗时间的震惊和痛苦之情,以及卫生部部长Jeremy Hunt对事件的相关处理。

【解题思路】

36. C　第三段"it is estimated between 135 and 270 women had their lives shortened as a result.",据估计,135至270名女性因为乳腺癌筛查出现错误,导致了寿命缩短。

37. C　第五段"He said he was watching the television on Wednesday when the news of the screening error broke, leaving him 'shell shocked'.",可知,乳腺癌筛查出现错误使Brian Gough感到吃惊。

38. D　原文并未提及所有的女性被邀请去做筛查。因此,D选项为错误选项,故选D。

39. B　文章十二段"It does seem strange that people didn't come forward who were expecting to be invited and didn't get an invitation and that didn't set hares running, so that's one of the things we need to look at.",表明,Mr. Hunt想要弄清楚为什么人们没有被邀请去做检查。

40. D　文章倒数第四段和第五段提到了chemotherapy, radiotherapy/But he said it returned again, prompting another two years of chemotherapy and treatment during what he described as an "horrendous situation",表明Gough的妻子接受了化疗,从Gough对化疗过程的描述,可以推测Gough的妻子经历了痛苦的治疗过程。

41. C　文中最后一段"Mr. Gough believes that 'maybe, just maybe' his wife might have come through the first lot of cancer treatment and survived if it had been diagnosed earlier." 可知,Gough假设疾病如果早点被诊断出来,他的妻子可能会幸存,而C项表述过于肯定。

42. B　文章讲述了Gough对于自己的妻子因为乳腺癌筛查出现错误,而错失最佳治疗时间的震惊和痛苦之情。因此,B选项的内容适合做文章的标题。

Part Three

【文章大意】文章介绍了神经性厌食症和贪食症,以及给出了相应的治疗建议。

【解题思路】

43. A　根据第一段"Most people know about anorexia nervous—when people deliberately starve themselves to keep their weight down—but bulimia, or excessive

vomiting, is another extreme of the disorder. ",题目正确。

44. A 根据第四段"They delude themselves into thinking that the only way to keep the calories they have eaten from turning into fat is to make themselves vomit or by taking excessive amounts of laxatives. ",题目正确。

45. A 根据第六段"It isn't just women who can suffer from anorexia or bulimia, although women are 10 times more liable to succumb to eating disorders. ",可知"女性比男性更容易饮食失调",所以题目正确,选 A。

46. B 根据第八段第一句"The frequent food binges by bulimics can lead to depression. ",频繁地大吃大喝能够导致抑郁,但并不是抑郁的直接原因,所以题目错误。

47. A 根据第九段"One of the obvious signs of bulimia is hard skin or marks on the back of the hand due to repeated abrasion of the skin as the hand is thrust down the throat to produce vomiting. ",题目正确。

48. B 根据倒数第四段"A sympathetic ear is the first priority when it comes to treating the disorder. ",当治疗这种饮食失调时,富有同情心的倾听是优先考虑的,但并不是说它能治愈饮食失调,所以题目错误。

49. C 题目译为"营养学家能帮助治疗厌食症与暴食症,因为他们可以在如何健康饮食方面给予意见",此信息在文中没有给出,故选 C。

50. A 根据最后一段"There is help out there for anorexics and bulimics, but they must take the first step and seek help from their doctors as soon as possible before they seriously damage their health. ",题目正确。

Part Four

【文章大意】文章介绍了反式脂肪酸的定义、用途、坏处,以及对如何摄取脂肪给出建议。

【解题思路】

51. D 第三段介绍了反式脂肪的坏处。第一句指出反式脂肪会提高胆固醇,降低身体所需的好胆固醇。第二句高脂肪食品不仅仅会导致肥胖。因此本句选 D 项:"Trans fats build up in the body and block blood flow to the heart",译为"体内的反式脂肪堆积并阻止血液流向心脏",为合理选项。有助于正确选题的重要词句包括:raise bad cholesterol/lower the good cholesterol/cause obesity/at risk of developing heart disease or having a stroke。

52. F 第四段第一句介绍了什么是反式脂肪酸。第二句指出食品公司和餐馆选择使用反式脂肪的原因——它们很便宜,由它们制作的食物像饼干和烘焙食品的保质期更长。此处选 F 项:"They also improve the taste and texture of food. ",译为"它们还能改善食物的味道和质地"。这也是在说明反式脂肪酸在制作食物上的作用,承接上文,因此为合理选项。有助于正确选题的重要词句包括:they're cheap and they make food like crackers and baked goods last longer。

53. B 第五段第二句、第三句介绍了美国和加拿大这样的国家,政府对食品生产有新的限制,食品和饮料生产商必须在产品上贴上营养标签。此处选 B 项:"These list daily recommendations and detail all the ingredients in a product, including trans fats if they're

used.",译为"这些产品列出了每日建议,并详细介绍了产品中的所有成分,包括使用的反式脂肪酸"。此句承接上句,介绍标签上的具体内容,句意合理。有助于正确选题的重要词句包括：new government restrictions on food production/attach a Nutrition Fact label.

54. E　第六段第二句指出医生建议我们从不饱和脂肪中获取大部分脂肪卡路里。空格的下文指出：另一种方法是避免外出就餐,尤其是快餐店。此外,在生鲜部购买大多数你需要的食物,并且需要限制加工和包装食品的数量。由此表明,上文的内容在讲如何正确地摄取脂肪卡路里,因此此处选 E 项："Reading the list of ingredients on the label is a good way of avoiding dangerous ingredients like trans fats."译为"阅读标签上的配料清单是避免危险成分如反式脂肪的好方法",为合理选项。有助于正确选题的重要词句包括：get most of our fatty calories from unsaturated fats/avoid eating out/buy the majority of your food in the fresh-food section and limit the amount of processed and packaged food you buy.

55. C　第六段倒数第二句话译为"如果你年轻,你可能不认为这很重要,但是你现在做出的选择会影响你的余生"。此处选 C 项："The healthier your diet is now, the longer and healthier your life will be.",译为"你现在的饮食越健康,你的寿命越长,越健康"。承接上文,因此为合理选项。有助于正确选题的重要词句包括：You might not think this is important if you're young, but the choices you make now will affect you for the rest of your life.

Part Five

【文章大意】文章介绍了夜间痛性痉挛(夜间抽筋)的症状及一些治疗建议。

【解题思路】

56. A　此处句意为：即使是最健康的人也可能在紧张的一天之后腿部短促疼痛,选 A 符合语句逻辑。

57. B　"If this sort of night cramp becomes a real nuisance, avoiding over-stretching and taking tablets containing quinine sulphate at bed-time may be all that is needed."此句意思："如果这种夜间抽筋成为一种真正的麻烦,避免过度拉伸和在睡前服用含硫酸奎宁的药片也许就够了。"选 B 句意合理。

58. A　"A very small number of patients, however, cannot take quinine without becoming dizzy or getting buzzing in the ears."此处句意为："然而,有少数患者服用奎宁会晕眩或耳朵嗡嗡作响。"选 A：引起头晕的,符合句意。B. lazy：懒惰的；C. crazy：疯狂的；D. fuzzy：模糊的。

59. C　"But cramp in the lower limbs in the daytime and in younger, active patients can be very distressing and is more serious."此句意思："然而,白天下肢抽筋以及年轻活跃的病人抽筋可能会非常痛苦并且更加严重。"故选 C。

60. D　"The patient first complains of aching legs after exercise. It may be slight, but gradually becomes more pronounced."此处句意为："病人首先主诉运动后腿痛。它可能是轻微的,但逐渐变得更加明显。"选 D：明显的,符合句意。

61. C　"Then the pain is not merely an ache, but a definite, crippling cramp, which can become so severe that the patient finds he or she cannot stand after much walking."此句表明这种痉挛性抽筋的疼痛在病人长时间行走之后会变得很严重,所以病人无法站立,

选 C 符合语句逻辑。

62. B "It generally means that the arteries everywhere in the body have become narrowed and blood cannot reach the muscles fast enough when they are in use. The heart muscles may be equally affected."此处译为："它通常意味着身体周围的动脉已经变窄,血液不能快速到达肌肉。"所以可以判断,心肌可能也同样受到了影响。选其他选项句子意义均不符合常理或逻辑。

63. A In a draught 意为"在风口",故选 A 项,符合句意。

64. B "The patient learns to regulate the amount of exercise he or she can comfortably take."此句意思:"病人学会调节自身运动量,以舒适为度。"选 B:调节,符合句意。

65. D "No drugs offer a complete relief but there is one habit which the sufferer must give up—smoking."此句句意为:没有药物能完全缓解,但有一种习惯必须让患者必须放弃——吸烟。选 D:放弃,句意合理。A. give out:分发 B. give back:归还 C. give away:赠送。

Ⅲ Writing

66.【范文】

Recent decades have witnessed the rapid development of medical and health system in China. Medical and health standards, in both metropolis and rural areas, have been significantly enhanced. However, we can not deny that some problems emerged in the meantime. Therefore, medical reform is imperative.

What problems need prompt solutions? First, uneven distribution of medical resources is a burning issue. According to the statistics released in 2018, the number of third-class hospitals in developed areas are almost as many as three times of those in underdeveloped areas. What's more, it is reported that most medical students look forward to working in hospitals in big cities after graduation, which further results in an uneven distribution of doctors. Second, high drug price is another problem crying for solution. Though some medicine can be paid by Medicare, some newly developed medicine, fairly expensive, are not included in Medicare. For example, patients feel desperate if they are diagnosed with cancer, because they cannot afford the treatment even after selling all their possessions.

To solve the above problems, the government should attract more medical talents to work in relatively underdeveloped areas by properly enhancing their welfare, and measures to encourage medical research such as increasing funds should be taken. (204 words)

【审题】

写作部分要求围绕"中国医疗改革"进行写作,要求分析目前我国医疗体系存在的问题,并给出自己对医疗改革的建议。文章应属说明文,写作的第一个重点是针对存在的问题,给出有针对性的具体建议。第二个重点是正确写出一些涉及医疗卫生领域话题的英语表达,如"医疗资源、三甲医院、医疗保险"等。

【范文评析】

　　文章首先陈述了近几十年来我国医疗卫生事业的发展,随后转折,指出目前仍存在问题,医疗改革刻不容缓。文章的重点放在问题的剖析上。第二段以问句开头,随后提出亟待解决的第一个问题,并列出数据展开论述。接着提出第二个亟须解决的问题,并通过具体事例展开论述。最后有针对性地提出两点建议。

　　文章语言表达准确,过渡自然,特别是第二段,并熟练运用"first""what is more""second"等表达引导观点陈述,运用"according to""for example"等表达引导论证。插入语的使用(in both metropolis and rural areas/fairly expensive)是本文句子水平上的一个亮点。

医护英语水平考试(三级)
模拟训练(七)

听力文本

This is METS-3 listening test. There are four parts in the test, Part One, Two, Three, and Four. You will hear each part twice. We will now stop for a moment before we start the test. Please ask any questions now because you must not speak during the test. Now, look at the instructions for Part One.

You will hear five extracts from conversations taking place in different clinical departments. Choose which case each doctor is discussing from the list A—F. Use each letter A—F only once. There is one extra letter which you do not need to use. Mark the corresponding letter on your answer sheet. You will hear each extract twice. Now we are ready to start.

Extract 1

Congratulations! Now your calcium level has improved and you can leave the hospital. But don't forget that your previous pathology report showed an adenoma of the abnormal gland. On your first postoperative day, you complained of perioral numbness and tingling, and your serum calcium was subnormal. Pay attention to your diet!

Extract 2

I suggest you try an insulin pump to give yourself more freedom and enhance your quality of life. It is about the size of a beeper with a thin catheter that you can introduce through a needle into your abdominal subcutaneous tissue. You can administer your insulin in a continuous subcutaneous insulin infusion and in calculated meal bolus doses. Of course you still have to test your blood for hyperglycemia and hypoglycemia and your urine for ketones when your blood sugar is too high.

Extract 3

Your daughter is diagnosed with pneumonia. You said she has been very lethargic, had a fever of 104°F, and has had muscular rigidity for 3 days. Actually, she took Haldol and Cogentin. Her secondary diagnosis is stated as neuroleptic malignant syndrome, a rare and life-threatening disorder associated with the use of antipsychotic medications.

Extract 4

You have been scheduled for surgery for a cataract and relief from "floaters". You should report to the ambulatory surgery center an hour before your scheduled procedure. Before transfer to the operating room, you'd better speak with your ophthalmologist and review the surgical plan.

Extract 5

I am sorry that your boy has osteogenesis imperfecta type III. His congenital disease is manifested by a defect in the creation of bone matrix, which gives normal bone its strength. His bones are very brittle and broken with little pressure or trauma. He also has a pectus cavernosus of his chest, an inversion or concavity of the sternum.

Now you'll hear Part One again. This is the end of Part One. Now look at Part Two.
You will hear a conversation between a reporter and a hair restoration expert. For each of the following statements, decide whether it is True (A) or False (B). If there is not enough information to answer True (A) or False (B), choose Not Given (C). Mark the corresponding letter on your answer sheet. You will hear the recording twice.

Reporter: I am Ann Lynn. It is reported that as many as half of all women are affected by hair loss at some time in their lives. I am interviewing Lisa Ishii, a Johns Hopkins hair restoration expert. She will answer questions about hair loss. Hi, Dr. Ishii, why many women lose hair?

Ishii: There are several factors that may cause hair loss. Women, most commonly, begin losing hair as a part of the normal aging process, but for others, it can be caused by hormone changes, medications taken for other purposes or severe, extreme stress.

Reporter: How does hair loss differ between men and women?

Ishii: There are a number of reasons for hair loss, but women go through unique hormone changes that contribute to specific types of female hair loss. For example, you may experience hair loss after going through pregnancy or if you have polycystic ovary syndrome. Hair loss patterns also vary between men and women. Men tend to see hair loss start at the temples, the hairline in an M shape and in the crown area, or we say, the "bald spot". As a woman, you may see hair thinning at the top of your head while your hairline remains intact, or you might notice a Christmas tree shape forming as the part of your hair becomes wider, a common symptom in female pattern hair loss.

Reporter: When it is necessary to talk to a doctor about hair loss?

Ishii: For women who are concerned about changes in their hair, there is never a bad time to talk to a doctor. If there is a sudden onset of hair loss, it is important to talk to a doctor to identify the root cause. If there is a noticeable change in the density of hair or if the hair is falling out in clumps, it is also necessary to see a care provider.

Reporter: Is there anything we can do at home to reduce hair loss and regrow hair?

Ishii: For the most common type of hair loss and genetic alopecia, I recommend hair treatments containing minoxidil, an FDA-approved medication for treatment of hair loss that is available over the counter.

Reporter: What are treatment options for hair loss?

Ishii: Depending on the cause of hair loss, there are several treatment options available to women. Some doctors may prescribe new medications, such as minoxidil and finasteride. Hair transplantation is also a viable option for many women. In this treatment, hair roots from the back and sides of the scalp are moved to the area we are trying to make more hair dense. The procedure takes several hours to complete, depending on the number of hair roots, and can be performed under light sedation or local anesthesia. New hair growth occurs in as little as four months, but multiple sessions may be required to achieve the desired effect.

Now you'll hear Part Two again. This is the end of Part Two. Now look at Part Three. You will hear a discussion among an instructor and two medical students. For questions 14—20, choose the most appropriate answer. Mark the corresponding letter on your answer sheet. You will hear the discussion twice.

Instructor: Today we are going to discuss the MRI navigational technology. The new treatment, carried out by neurosurgeons at the UCSD School of Medicine and the UCSD Moores Cancer Center, uses real-time MRI, that is, magnetic resonance imaging as a way of guiding the delivery of the new gene therapy directly into brain tumors.

Student 1: How does the MRI guided gene therapy work? Previous efforts with gene therapy for brain cancer were largely limited by the inability to deliver the drug into the brain. Under normal conditions, the brain is protected by a physiological system called the blood-brain barrier.

Student 2: This natural defense mechanism also prevents drugs from reaching the cancer cells in brain tumor patients. It is estimated that less than 1% of all available drugs will cross the blood brain barrier.

Instructor: Right. In the new treatment, the blood brain barrier is by-passed by directly injecting the gene therapy into the region of the tumor. To ensure that the adequate amount of agent is delivered to the region of the tumor, a state-of-the-art MRI technology is utilized to monitor the delivery and injection processes in real time. The MRI-guided process provides visual confirmation that adequate amount of the therapy is delivered into the tumor. Additionally, the ability to visualize the delivery catheter in real-time prevents any unintended injury to the brain.

Student 1: What are the benefits and risks of using this treatment?

Instructor: To understand the benefits of the therapy, we first need to review the basis of the gene therapy. The gene therapy is based on a retro-virus engineered to selectively replicate in high grade brain cancer cells. This virus produces an enzyme that converts the FDA approved anti-fungal drug flucytosine, or 5 - FC into the anti-cancer drug 5-fluorouracil, or 5 - FU. After the injection of the virus, the patients are treated with oral formulations of 5 - FC. Tumor kill is induced when 5 - FC comes into contact with cells infected with virus.

Student 2: Typically, when chemotherapy is given, just about every cell in the body is exposed to the potential side-effects of the drug. The direct injection approach limits the presence of the active drug in the brain tumor and not elsewhere in the body. Consequently, the approach protects the patient from many of the intended side-effects of chemotherapy.

Instructor: The virus has been tested in a large number of patients and has been shown to be safe. So the risks of the treatment relates to the surgical procedure itself. The MRI technology allows the surgeon to visualize the delivery catheter in real-time. In doing so, the surgeon can prevent any unintended injury to the brain during the procedure. So, the risk of the procedure is lowered to an absolute minimum.

Now you'll hear Part Three again. This is the end of Part Three. Now look at Part Four. You will hear a speech on diets helping some people with Hashimoto's disease. Complete the notes. In each blank, write only one word. Write the answers on your answer sheet. You will hear the speech twice.

Male: Hashimoto's disease is the most common autoimmune condition and the leading cause of hypothyroidism. It is sometimes called Hashimoto's thyroiditis or shortened to Hashimoto's.

The thyroid gland plays a major role in metabolism, hormone regulation, and body temperature. When a person has Hashimoto's, his/her thyroid is chronically inflamed and cannot function as well as a healthy thyroid. The thyroid often slows or stops the production of essential hormones, which can cause weight gain, dry skin, hair loss, fatigue, constipation, and sensitivity to cold.

There is no specific diet proven to treat everyone with Hashimoto's. An individualized approach to nutrition is necessary.

Some clinical evidence has shown that the following diets have helped some people with Hashimoto's, which are gluten-free diet, grain-free diet, paleo diet and nutrient-dense diet. Now, we take a closer look at some of these diets.

First, gluten-free diet. Many people with Hashimoto's also experience food sensitivities, especially to gluten. There is no current research to support a gluten-free diet for all people with Hashimoto's unless they also have celiac disease. Gluten-free diets remove all foods with containing gluten, which is a protein found in wheat, barley, rye, and other grains. Gluten is commonly found in pasta, bread, baked goods, beer, soups, and cereals. The best way to go gluten-free is to focus on foods that are naturally gluten-free, such as vegetables, fruits, lean meats, seafood, beans, legumes, nuts, and eggs.

Second, grain-free diet. A grain-free diet is very similar to gluten-free, except that grains are also off-limits. These grains include amaranth, teff, quinoa, millet, oats and buckwheat. There is little evidence, however, that cutting out non-gluten grains is beneficial for health. Cutting out these grains may also eliminate fiber and other sources of essential nutrients, such as selenium, which are important for people with Hashimoto's.

Third, paleo diet. The paleo diet attempts to mimic the eating patterns of our early ancestors, with an emphasis on whole, unprocessed foods. Grains, dairy, potatoes, beans, lentils, refined sugar, and refined oils are not allowed. Cage-free and grass-fed meats are encouraged, as are vegetables, nuts (except peanuts), seeds, seafood, and healthful fats, such as avocado and olive oil.

Fourth, nutrient-dense diet. For people who do not want to focus on what foods to cut out, opting for a nutrient-dense diet plan may be the best option. A nutrient-dense diet includes variety and focuses on whole foods with a selection of colorful fruits and vegetables, healthy fats, lean proteins, and fibrous carbohydrates. Foods include leafy greens, fatty fish, a variety of colored vegetables, fruits, healthful fats, lean proteins, fibrous foods. Having these foods as the primary focus of the diet will leave less room for processed and refined sugar foods. Anti-inflammatory spices such as turmeric, ginger, and garlic are also encouraged.

It is more important for a person to follow a well-balanced diet that works for their lifestyle than to try to put a label on their eating habits. People should focus on whole, unprocessed foods and eat foods that grow in the ground, not foods that come in a box or a bag.

People with Hashimoto's should be open to trying different eating styles until they find the one that makes them feel best. They should also speak to a doctor or dietitian about how to make sure they get all of the essential nutrients.

Now you'll hear Part Four again. This is the end of Part Four. You now have five minutes to write your answers on the answer sheet. You have one more minute. This is the end of the listening test.

参考答案与试题评析

Ⅰ Listening

Part One

1.【语段大意】医生祝贺患者钙水平提高,可以出院,但提醒患者曾经的病理报告显示腺瘤,且术后第一天口周有麻木和刺痛感,提醒患者注意饮食。

【解题思路】A 听力开始部分可听到 Now your calcium level has improved and you can leave the hospital 这一关键信息。

2.【语段大意】医生建议患者尝试使用胰岛素泵,并介绍了使用方法。

【解题思路】D 可听到 try an insulin pump, administer your insulin 等关键信息。

3.【语段大意】医生告知,患者被诊断为患有肺炎和神经阻滞剂恶性综合征(neuroleptic malignant syndrome)。

【解题思路】C 可听到 Your daughter is diagnosed with pneumonia, Her secondary diagnosis is stated as neuroleptic malignant syndrome 等关键信息。

4.【语段大意】患者已被安排白内障手术,工作人员建议患者在手术前一小时到门诊手术中心报告,并最好在手术前与眼科医生谈一谈。

【解题思路】E 可听到 cataract, ophthalmologist 等关键词。

5.【语段大意】医生告知患者家属,孩子患有Ⅲ型成骨不全(osteogenesis imperfecta type Ⅲ),骨骼脆弱。

【解题思路】F 可听到 His bones are very brittle 这一关键句。

Part Two

【语篇大意】一位记者对一位植发专家的采访。

【解题思路】

6. A 专家提到开始脱发是女性正常衰老过程的一部分,故答案为 A。

7. A 专家提到脱发有很多原因,但女性会经历独特的荷尔蒙变化而导致特定类型的脱发。故答案为 A。

8. C 专家举例说,女性怀孕或患有多囊卵巢综合征(polycystic ovary syndrome)会导致脱发，未提及生产与脱发有关联，所以答案为 C。

9. A　专家提到男性倾向于从太阳穴（temple）开始脱发，所以 A 正确。

10. A　专家提到，如果突然出现脱发，应去看医生，找出根本原因，因此选 A。

11. A　对于最常见的脱发和遗传性脱发（genetic alopecia），专家推荐使用含有米诺地尔（minoxidil）的药物，此药物是 FDA 批准的治疗脱发的非处方药，所以选 A。

12. B　专家提到，植发是女性的可行性选择，所以选 B。

13. B　听力最后部分提到，新发生长最少需四个月，故 B 正确。

Part Three

【语篇大意】两位医学生与老师讨论磁共振导航技术（MRI navigational technology）的相关问题。

【解题思路】

14. A　对话中提到，以前对脑肿瘤进行基因治疗的限制，很大程度上在于无法将药物输送到大脑。故答案为 A。关键信息：Previous efforts with gene therapy for brain cancer were largely limited by the inability to deliver the drug into the brain.

15. B　一个学生提到，在正常情况下，大脑受到一种叫做血脑屏障（blood-brain barrier）的生理系统的保护。接着另一个学生补充说，这种天然防御机制也阻止药物到达脑肿瘤患者的癌细胞。故答案为 B。关键信息：Under normal conditions, the brain is protected by a physiological system called the blood-brain barrier. /This natural defense mechanism also prevents drugs from reaching the cancer cells in brain tumor patients.

16. B　对话中提到，在新疗法中，通过直接注射基因进入肿瘤区，绕开了血脑屏障。所以答案应该选 B。关键信息：In the new treatment, the blood brain barrier is by-passed by directly injecting the gene therapy into the region of the tumor.

17. C　MRI 引导下，治疗传送过程是可视的。故答案为 C。关键信息：The MRI-guided process provides visual confirmation that adequate amount of the therapy is delivered into the tumor.

18. A　对话中提到基因治疗的基础是一种逆转录病毒，B 是化疗，C 是水疗，显然 A 正确。关键信息：The gene therapy is based on a retro-virus engineered to selectively replicate in high grade brain cancer cells.

19. A　对话中提到，在通常情况下，化疗的潜在副作用会影响到体内几乎所有细胞。故答案为 A。关键信息：Typically, when chemotherapy is given, just about every cell in the body is exposed to the potential side-effects of the drug.

20. C　对话中提到治疗的风险与手术有关。故答案为 C。关键信息：So the risks of the treatment relates to the surgical procedure itself.

Part Four

【语篇大意】关于淋巴细胞性甲状腺肿（Hashimoto's disease）的一段讲座。

【解题思路】

21. hypothyroidism　讲座一开始提到，淋巴细胞性甲状腺肿是最常见的自身免疫性疾病，也是甲状腺功能减退（hypothyroidism）的主要原因。所以此处应填 hypothyroidism。

22. protein　此处为讲座中提到的第一种能帮助淋巴细胞性甲状腺肿患者的饮食，即无麸质饮食(gluten-free diets),麸质是一种在小麦、大麦、黑麦和其他谷物中发现的蛋白质。所以此处应填 protein。

23. unprocessed　此处为讲座中提到的第三种能帮助淋巴细胞性甲状腺肿患者的饮食,即古旧饮食(paleo diet)。古旧饮食试图模仿我们早期祖先的饮食模式,关键在于完整的、且未加工的食物。所以此处应填 unprocessed。

24. Anti-inflammatory　此处为讲座中提到的第四种能帮助淋巴细胞性甲状腺肿患者的饮食,即 nutrient-dense diet(营养密集型膳食)。此部分最后提到,有抗炎作用的调味品,如姜黄、生姜和大蒜等,也鼓励食用。所以此处应填 anti-inflammatory。

25. well-balanced　此处为讲座总结部分,遵循平衡饮食的生活方式比把自己的饮食习惯贴上标签更为重要。故此处应填 well-balanced。

Ⅱ　Reading

Part One

【文章大意】文章通过研究表明低盐饮食并不适合每一个人,同时介绍了一些国家食盐量的情况。

【解题思路】

26. C　根据第一段第一、第二句"Low-salt diets are actually harmful to our bodies, a recent study found. These diets may actually increase the risk of developing heart disease, or even cause death."直接指出:最近的一项研究表明低盐饮食可能会增加患心脏病,甚至猝死的风险。

27. A　第二段第一句介绍本次研究人员的身份;第二句介绍研究对象和方法;第三句介绍研究目的;第四句为研究结果;第五、第六句是本次研究提出的建议。

28. E　第三段开头"This study adds to our understanding of the relationship between salt intake and health. The study also questions the correctness of present guidelines that recommend low salt intake for everyone."和第三段倒数第三句"Mente added that the current general recommendations relating to the maximum healthy salt intake seems too low, especially since they do not consider an individual's blood pressure.",表明,O'Donnell 和 Mente 对当前健康盐摄入量的准则和建议进行了质疑和否定。

29. B　第四段第一、第二句第三句指出世界上大多数人对钠的摄入量是健康的,即每天不超过 6 克;但是第四句指出对一些易患高血压人群以及高盐人群应降低盐摄入量;第五句作者表示不认同当前许多国家的关于降低钠摄入量的指导方法。

30. D　第五段列举加拿大、美国和肯尼亚三国对不同人群提出的盐摄入量指导标准进行描述。

31. E　定位第一段第三句"These findings, says WebMD, a public health website, are contrary to the popular wisdom that has long said low-salt diets are healthy."。

32. D　定位第二段倒数第二句"The study goes on to suggest that only certain people should be concerned about reducing sodium in their diets."。

33. B　定位第三段第二句"The study also questions the correctness of present guidelines that recommend low salt intake for everyone."。

34. F 定位第三段第二句"Mente does not agree with the current strategy of reducing sodium intake in almost all countries."。

35. A 定位第五段第四句"For those over 51 and persons of any age who are African American or have hypertension, diabetes, or chronic kidney disease, the US guidelines suggest having less than 1.5 grams a day."。

Part Two

【文章大意】主要介绍病人病史的几个组成部分。

【解题思路】

36. D 第一段第二句"On the other hand, a poorly documented history and physical exam may lead to confusion, serious omission of vital data and inefficiency on patient rounds."指写得差的病史记录和体检会导致的三个结果,D 选项不是其结果。

37. D 在对"Identification"表述的段落中"The patient's name written in the history allows future interviewers to address the patient by his name which conveys a sense of patient respect. The age, race, sex and occupation are important as many diseases are not only gender and age dependent, but may also occur more commonly in specific ethnic and occupation groups.",提到了身份认同的重要性,A、B、C 选项都符合,故选 D。

38. C A、B、D 选项中关于既往病史、病人主诉以及病人的职业、性别、性行为和非法药物使用的内容在文章中都有相关表述,C 选项 Treatment Plan 在最后一段提及,但治疗计划并不包含于病史之中。

39. B 文章在论述"Chief Complaint"时,第一句话"This should be written in the patient's words.",可知,病人主诉应该用病人的言语来表达,而非医生的经验。

40. B "ROS（Review of Systems）—This section is too often omitted. Social History—This section is the most neglected section of the patient history performed in China."表明,系统回顾与社交史都是病史中容易忽略的部分,社交史在中国病人病史中是最容易被忽略的,因此 B 选项的表述是错误的。

41. A 最后一段中的"rapport"意思是关系,在原文指的是医患之间的良好关系,因此 A 选项为正确选项。

42. C 本题为主旨题。文章主要介绍病人病史的几个组成部分,最后一段总结了病人病史的作用,所以,文章的写作意图是强调病人病史的重要性,故选 C 选项。

Part Three

【文章大意】文章讨论了咖啡与健康的关系,尤其探讨了饮用咖啡是否会致癌。

【解题思路】

43. A 根据第一段"Trouble is brewing for coffee lovers in California, where a judge ruled that sellers must post scary warnings about cancer risks. But how frightened should we be of a daily cup of coffee? Not very, some scientists and available evidence seem to suggest.",题目正确。

44. A 根据第二段第一句"Scientific concerns about coffee have eased in recent years, and many studies even suggest it can help health.",题目正确。

45. A 根据第三段"CBS News medical contributor Dr. David Agus, director of the

Westside Cancer Center at USC，says he believes it is too early to put this kind of blanket warning on coffee. "以及第四段"to me it causes panic rather than informed knowledge"，可知,Dr. David Agus 认为贴警示会导致恐慌。

46. C　题目大意为世界卫生组织已经做好计划来预防癌症可能的风险,此信息在文中没有给出,故选 C。

47. B　根据第六段"The current flap isn't about coffee itself，but a chemical called acrylamide that's made when the beans are roasted. Government agencies call it a probable or likely carcinogen，based on animal research"，当豆子烤好的时候，一种叫做丙烯酰胺的化学物质产生了。政府机构基于动物研究的基础上,认为这种化学物质可能致癌,因此题目错误。

48. A　根据第八段"'A cup of coffee a day，exposure probably is not that high,' and probably should not change your habit，said Dr. Bruce Y. Lee of Johns Hopkins Bloomberg School of Public Health. 'If you drink a lot of cups a day，this is one of the reasons you might consider cutting that down. '"表明,每天喝咖啡要适度,所以题目正确。

49. C　倒数第二段第一句"Start with the biggest known risk factor for cancer—smoking—which generates acrylamide. "，吸烟是患癌风险最大的因素,但原文没有提及吸烟可以导致肺癌,故选 C。

50. B　最后一段"A group of 23 scientists convened by the WHO's cancer agency in 2016 looked at coffee—not acrylamide directly—and decided coffee was unlikely to cause breast，prostate or pancreatic cancer，and that it seemed to lower the risks for liver and uterine cancers. "表明,参会专家认为咖啡不太可能引起乳腺癌、前列腺癌或胰腺癌,所以题目错误。

Part Four
【文章大意】文章介绍了一种新药,老鼠使用这种药物后,会带来和运动相同的益处。但不久药物出现问题,人未使用。但研究者一直研发类似但不会对人体造成危害的药物。同时,体育界很多人都担心运动员使用这样的药丸。

【解题思路】
51. D　第一段开头介绍药丸可以解决很多问题。随后第五句"But what about people who are overweight or lack fitness?"(但是超重或缺乏健康的人怎么办呢?)D 项:"The best solution for these people is to exercise，but many people don't want to exercise or are unable to exercise. "(对这些人最好的解决办法是锻炼身体,但很多人不想锻炼或不能锻炼。)恰好回答了上文中提出的问题,因此为合理选项。有助于正确选题的重要词句包括:But what about people who are overweight or lack fitness?

52. E　第二段开头介绍了老鼠使用药物后的良好效果,以及不久后出现的问题。E 项:"Researchers found that mice had an increased chance of developing cancer after taking it. "(研究人员发现,小鼠服药后患癌症的概率增加了。)承接上文,为合理选项。有助于正确选题的重要词句包括:reports about problems with the drug soon began appearing. /This meant the drug would never be approved for human use.

53. B　第三段首句介绍医学研究人员仍在寻找类似于 90 年代发现的药物,上文提到该药会导致癌症。B项:"They're trying to find a new drug with the same benefits that doesn't also cause cancer."(他们试图找到一种具有相同药效但不会导致癌症的新药物。)下文也提到了此药会有很多用途,所以选项符合句意表达,为合理选项。有助于正确选题的重要词句包括:looking for a drug similar to the one found in the 90s. /They believe such a drug would have many uses.

54. A 该空的上一句话讲该药有利于糖尿病患者和那些患有肌肉萎缩疾病的患者。下文也提到了很多成年人没时间做医生建议的运动量。A项:"Medical researchers also believe such a drug could benefit the average adult as well."(医学研究者也相信这种药物对普通成年人也有好处。)因此,A选项为合理选项。

55. F 第四段第二句和第三句句意为:"他们担心一些运动员可能会用它作为一种提高运动成绩的药物。即使在90年代发现的药物从来没有被批准用于人类,一些运动员可能会用它来作弊。"F项:"Many people in the world of sports are concerned about a pill like this."(体育界很多人都担心这样的药丸。)选项内容与下文内容相符,因此为合理选项。

Part Five

【文章大意】本文介绍了许多国家的肥胖问题,以及肥胖给人身体带来的风险。

【解题思路】

56. B 本文讲的内容为肥胖问题,根据句意理解,世界性的体重问题在发达国家和贫穷国家应该都在增长,故选B。

57. A 根据句意理解,越来越多的人死于和健康相关的问题,因此选A。related:相关的。

58. C "About four million people died of cardiovascular disease, diabetes, cancer and other diseases linked to excess weight in 2015, according to the study."此句意为:"根据这项研究,2015年,大约有四百万人死于心血管疾病、糖尿病、癌症和其他与超重有关的疾病。"选C:超重的,符合句意。extra:额外的;extensive:广泛的;undue:过分的。

59. D "They examined obesity rates, average weight gain and the cause of death in 195 countries."上句提到研究者研究了从1980年到2015年的健康信息,所以此句的句意是"他们调查了195个国家的肥胖率、平均体重增加和死亡原因"。故选examined:调查,仔细检查;其他选项不符合句意。

60. A 下文提到了埃及、越南、美国以及孟加拉国,这几个国家都是人口众多的国家,故选A. populous:人口众多的。此句句意为"2015年人口数在前20的国家中"。

61. D "Researchers say the extra weight people are carrying increases their risk of developing diabetes or other health problems."此句意为:"研究人员表示,人们额外增加的体重增加了患糖尿病或其他健康问题的风险。"选D:developing 患(病),符合句意。

62. C 根据下文理解,此处为转折。故选C. Yet:然而。

63. A "Experts said poor diets and lack of physical activity are mainly to blame for the rising numbers of overweight people."此句意为:"专家说超重的人数不断增加归咎于饮食不好和缺乏体育锻炼。"因此选A. blame for:归咎于。B. scold:责骂;C. condemn:谴责;D. charge:指控。

64. B "Growing populations have brought about rising obesity rates in poor

countries. "此句句意为:"不断增长的人口导致贫困国家的肥胖率不断上升。"B. brought about:导致,符合句意。A. resulted from:起因于;C. attributed to:归因于;D. given out:分发。

65. C "It found that the cost of processed foods like ice cream and hamburgers has fallen since 1990. But the cost of fresh fruits and vegetables has gone up. "此处下句句意为"新鲜水果和蔬菜的价格上涨了",而且上下文是转折关系,所以,此句的意思为:"研究发现,自 1990 以来,加工食品如冰激淋和汉堡包的成本有所下降。"故选 C. fallen:下降。

Ⅲ Writing

66.【范文】

With the rapid development of society, modern people have been paying great attention to leading a healthy life. Though it has been generally accepted that sports play a vital role in physical health, some claim that many diseases are actually caused by emotional management failure.

There is no doubt that doing regular exercises is of great importance in living a healthy life. As many medical researches point out, aerobic exercises are conducive to the heart and lungs, and are beneficial to the blood circulation system, the respiratory system and the digestive system. Doing physical exercises regularly can reduce the risks of many death-causing diseases such as heart disease, high blood pressure and diabetes. In addition, physical exercise is an effective way to treat sub-health.

Nevertheless, emotional management is also crucial. As we all know, negative emotions such as sadness, fear and anger are potentially risky to health. The body changes in a number of ways under bad emotions: blood pressure and pulse rate rise, breathing becomes faster, the digestive system slows down, immune activity decreases, the muscles become rigid and a heightened state of alertness prevents sleep. Mental diseases such as psychiatric disorders and depression may be caused by long-term negative emotions. So keeping good mood is an effective way to keep healthy. It is not rare to hear that optimism can improve the cure rate of diseases.

In sum, to lead a healthy life, doing exercises and controlling emotions are of equal significance. (245 words)

【审题】

写作部分要求讨论运动和情绪管理对"健康生活"的重要性。文章应属议论文,应就题目给出的两个方面进行讨论,并给出自己的观点。写作中的一个重点和难点是如何正确写出一些涉及医疗卫生领域话题的英语表达,如"有氧运动、血液循环系统、呼吸系统、消化系统、心脏病、高血压、糖尿病、亚健康、精神疾病、抑郁症"等。

【范文评析】

文章采用四段式写作结构。第一段根据作文任务给定的信息展开讨论,段落中运用"though"这一表转折关系词汇陈述两种观点,用"it has been generally accepted"和"some claim"不同表达分述人们对两种观点的不同认知程度。第二段和第三段为主体部分。第二段第一句总领全段,以"there is no doubt"引入运动能带来的好处；随后第三段从正反两方面阐述了情绪对健康的影响。最后一段简明扼要地给出作者的观点。

　　文章论证充分,用详实的例子就健康的两个方面进行了讨论；语言表达多样(people pay great attention to health/is of great importance/crucial/are of equal significance)；熟练使用 as many medical researches point out，as we all know 等衔接手段。